MENOPAUSE SPOTLIGHT

Understanding and Managing Brain Fog

Menopause Spotlight

Understanding and Managing Brain Fog

R. D. Bennett

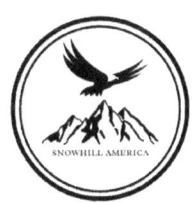

Copyright © 2025 by R.D. Bennett

All rights reserved.

Published by

Snowhill America

[www.snowhillamerica.com]

No part of this book may be reproduced, distributed, or transmitted in any form or by any means, including photocopying, recording, or other electronic or mechanical methods, without the prior written permission of the publisher, except in the case of brief quotations used in reviews, academic purposes, or as permitted by copyright law.

First Edition: 2024

Second Edition: 2025

ISBN: 979-8-9926797-2-4

The advice and strategies contained in this book are for informational purposes only. The author and publisher make no representations or warranties with respect to the accuracy or completeness of the contents and disclaim any implied warranties of fitness for a particular purpose. Readers should seek professional guidance specific to their circumstances.

Cover by germancreative

Previously published as *The Menopausal Woman's Short Guide to Brain Fog* **by R.D. Bennett.**

Contents

1: Unlocking Mental Clarity During Menopause 7

2: Unraveling The Mystery Of Brain Fog 13

3: The Ripple Effects Of Brain Fog 21

4: Understanding Your Brain During Menopause: A Deeper Look . 33

5: Cognitive Function: Understanding The Brain's Needs 39

6: Hormones And Brain Fog: The Missing Link? 47

7: HRT: Help Or Hindrance? 55

8: Fueling Mental Clarity 59

9: Balancing Mind And Body For Mental Clarity 69

10: Navigating The Emotional Journey Of Brain Fog 75

11: Finding Strength In Support 81

12: Thriving At Work Despite Brain Fog 85

13: A Clearer Path Ahead 91

14: The Brain Fog Toolkit 95

Thank You 99

Resources 101

Other Books By R. D. Bennett 122

About The Author 123

1

Unlocking Mental Clarity During Menopause

Most women, as they approach their mid-40s, are keenly aware that menopause looms ahead. Recently, it seems everyone is talking about menopause, on TV, on the radio, and on the internet, and everyone, even the men, seems to have an opinion now!

Millions of women experience the symptoms of menopause every day. We all know the image of the poor woman who, for one minute, is fine, sipping her coffee, chatting away to you, and then suddenly turns a bright red, and sweat drips down her face, appearing to melt before your very eyes. A hot flash, out of nowhere, like a tiny volcano, had erupted inside her body. *This woman is on fire.* She vigorously fans herself with whatever she can, grabbing a notebook, a folder, or last week's grocery receipt because *nothing* can cool the inferno raging inside her. "Is it hot in here or just me?" she asks. She undressed, hoping to cool the inferno inside that she was feeling. She is suddenly experiencing the equator at the height of summer. "I'm fine," she cries through gritted teeth when asked, though her hair, plastered to her forehead, screams otherwise. While some women may get off lightly with just a mild heating, others explode into a full personal volcano. It is debilitating and embarrassing, and my heart goes out to all women who experience this. However, this is not the only debilitating symptom of menopause.

Approximately 1.3 million women each year will reach menopause in the United States, with 80% experiencing the most common physical symptom of hot flashes and 25-30% experiencing the most debilitating severe form. In addition, 50% of women will experience vaginal dryness and 20-40% will suffer a drop in libido. But while the physical symptoms of menopause are grabbing the headlines, people only secretly discuss the hidden effects on mental health for fear of being labeled as crazy.

For some women, the only noticeable physical symptoms of menopause, aside from the absence of a menstrual period, are night sweats. Although night sweats disrupt and cause discomfort for women, they usually experience these symptoms privately, without outwardly signaling menopause to others. This invisibility can present its own set of challenges, as others may not recognize or understand the physical and emotional struggles that accompany this phase of life. Night sweats and other menopausal symptoms often hide their effects on mental health and brain function, as fluctuating hormone levels often cause them, can interrupt sleep and lead to fatigue, irritability, or difficulty concentrating during the day.

However, night sweats are not the only symptoms that can affect your cognitive function. Another widely experienced but little-discussed symptom of menopause is brain fog.

We all forget things sometimes; it's perfectly normal. "You're just having one of those days. It's like when you walk into a room and totally forget why you're there, or when you're looking for your phone... while it is in your hands. You laugh it off, but it suddenly feels like you are having more of "those days." They gradually become more frequent and harder to laugh off.

Then your work is affected. You forget some details of a project you have been working on, the reason for a meeting, and even what you discussed yesterday. There you are, surrounded by your smart, competent colleagues, staring at a blank notepad as someone asks for your input. You open your mouth, fully intending to deliver a thoughtful response, but... nothing. It's as though your thoughts have packed their bags and taken a vacation without notifying you. It isn't just your memory that's affected; your ability to focus, organize, and even find the right words in conversation seems to slip away. Tasks that once felt routine now seem monumental, and you question yourself: *Am I losing it?*

Turns out that no, you are not "losing it." We are simply experiencing one of the lesser-talked-about realities of menopause: brain fog.

Brain fog? What is brain fog, you may ask. Now, if you had told me years ago that menopause would not just mess with my body but would also turn my brain into a foggy maze, I probably would not have believed you. No one prepares you for this part of the journey.

We hear all about hot flashes, mood swings, and night sweats, but brain fog? Rarely. That's a curveball that no one warns you about.

Menopause brain fog refers to a common set of cognitive challenges experienced by many women during menopause, often associated with hormonal fluctuations. It can manifest as forgetfulness, difficulty concentrating, mental fatigue, and slowed problem-solving abilities. Everyday tasks, such as recalling names, staying focused, or expressing thoughts clearly, may feel more challenging, as if one is thinking through a dense mental haze.

Menopausal brain fog can make you feel deeply isolated and incredibly frustrated, leaving you questioning whether your struggles are unique or even real. But here's the truth: brain fog is a genuine experience with biological and hormonal underpinnings, and you are far from alone in facing it. Understanding this can help you approach yourself with the compassion and kindness you truly deserve during this phase of life.

If you are reading this, chances are that you've felt the effects of brain fog firsthand. Perhaps you've forgotten something important, like your best friend's birthday, for the first time in years. Perhaps you found it difficult to find the right word during a critical moment at work or stood in a grocery store aisle, staring blankly at your shopping list. Millions of women share these unsettling moments, although they rarely discuss them openly.

The good news is that you are not alone. Menopausal brain fog affects countless women, yet the silence surrounding it often intensifies the sense of isolation. By shedding light on these challenges, we can normalize the conversation and create a space where women feel seen, heard, and supported.

Millions of women cope with the symptoms of menopause every day, and while 80% suffer from hot flashes, approximately 60% of women report experiencing cognitive difficulties, such as brain fog, during menopause. This highlights how common these challenges are, even though they are often under-recognized or misunderstood.

Recognizing and addressing this aspect of menopause is important. The fact that we are talking about it is great. We should spread this message to prevent women from becoming the butt of jokes and to ensure that support is available when needed. For too long, women have suffered in silence.

I am not a doctor, therapist, or healthcare practitioner, just another woman walking through this journey of menopause alongside you. I hope that the insights and tips shared here will offer encouragement and practical guidance as you manage menopause and its associated challenges, like brain fog. Together, through understanding and self-compassion, we can tackle this phase with renewed confidence and resilience. Always remember, you're not alone, and there is a community of women who understand exactly what you're going through.

2

Unraveling The Mystery Of Brain Fog

If you have ever walked into a room only to forget why you went there or blanked completely on a colleague's name, congratulations, you have experienced brain fog. That frustrating, hazy feeling makes your mind feel like it's wrapped in cotton candy instead of firing on all cylinders.

Now, imagine that instead of occurring every so often, it occurs daily, hourly, even by the minute (or so it feels). Combine it with the mighty hot flashes, and suddenly, you feel you are losing your mind. If there are no other underlying explanations for these memory lapses, you may experience brain fog as one of the many symptoms of menopause. While it is not an official medical term, millions of women experience it as part of their menopausal journey.

Brain fog is not a medical condition, but a general term used often to describe the temporary symptoms like mental fuzziness, short-term forgetfulness, and or difficulty concentrating menopausal women experience. Around 23% of women might encounter alterations in their brain function, like brain fog, during menopause. These changes often occur during the early stages of perimenopause, when estrogen levels decline, and the frequency and intensity of periods fluctuate.

Short-term forgetfulness may appear as misplacing things, losing your train of thought, or struggling to recall words and names. Examples of which could include forgetting why you walked into a room or what you were about to say; struggling to recall names, dates, or simple facts; frequently misplacing everyday items like keys or your phone; searching for words mid-sentence or mixing them up entirely (saying "refrigerator" when you meant "microwave"); or struggling to keep up with fast-paced conversations.

Difficulty concentrating may cause you to feel like it is difficult to stay focused on a task or a conversation. Perhaps you are zoning out during conversations or meetings, losing track of tasks, or forgetting what you were doing midway through, making it hard to concentrate on detailed work or multitask effectively.

Brain fog isn't about losing intelligence or capability, it's more like your brain's Wi-Fi is running on one bar with no Wi-Fi booster available.

One report evaluated brain scans of several perimenopausal women and found their brain activity to be 25% lower than that of women not yet in perimenopause. These brain changes were determined to be usually temporary, often reversing a couple of years after reaching menopause, when a woman no longer has periods (typically between the ages of 45 and 55), and did not take into consideration other causes that could affect brain function such as lack of sleep because of night sweats. In addition, another separate study in India has also suggested that hormonal changes during menopause, particularly the decline in estrogen levels, can affect cognitive functions like memory, focus, and mental clarity.

The long-term SWAN (Study of Women's Health Across the Nation) research provided valuable insights into menopause and its effects on brain function. It highlighted those cognitive changes, such as memory difficulties and slower processing speed, are common during the menopause transition, with these changes often linked to hormonal fluctuations, particularly declining estrogen levels, which play a role in brain health.

Mental fuzziness can feel like navigating your thoughts through a dense and impenetrable cloud where clarity seems just out of reach. A sense of cognitive sluggishness often accompanies this sensation and diminished mental sharpness. For example, you may feel mentally "drained" or exhausted, even after completing tasks that would typically seem simple or routine. Problem-solving abilities may feel noticeably slower, making it challenging to approach issues with the efficiency or confidence you're used to.

Mental fuzziness can leave you feeling easily overwhelmed by an influx of information or the need to decide, no matter how small they may seem. The sheer act of processing multiple inputs at once can feel daunting, causing a cascade of frustration or self-doubt. Expressing your thoughts can also become a struggle, as you may find yourself tongue-tied, unsure of how to articulate your ideas, or groping for the right words to convey what you're thinking.

This experience, while frustrating, is not uncommon and can occur during times of stress or exhaustion, as well as during hormonal changes.

Many women feel embarrassed or hesitant to talk about brain fog because they fear being judged. Instead, you might downplay your struggles, thinking they are "no big deal" or you are just "not feeling like myself". By understanding what brain fog is during menopause, why it happens, and how it shows up in your life, you can take the first steps toward managing it.

Brain fog, because of menopause, can look different for everyone, so it's important to recognize these signs for what they are: a temporary phase caused by real biological changes, not a reflection of your intelligence or capabilities. Brain fog is very common during perimenopause, and overall, 60% of women will reportedly suffer from brain fog in their lives. In a study, brain fog was among the symptoms often cited by women when describing that they were "Not feeling like myself".

In addition, the effect of other menopausal symptoms, such as night sweats, can cause sleep disturbances that may also contribute to the effects of brain fog. The human brain relies on quality sleep to perform its many functions, from establishing memories to staying healthy. Sleep deprivation, also known as sleep fatigue, is a reduction of brain function resulting from poor-quality sleep. Lack of sufficient rest may also contribute to worsening or causing brain fog. Sleep deprivation significantly affects concentration, decision-making, and problem-solving skills. The effects of one night of poor sleep can be equivalent to the legal driving limit for being under the influence of alcohol.

Sleep deprivation can also impair the conversion of short-term memories into long-term memories. Memory consolidation is important for processing new information and learning. While we may forget many things during the day, a reduction in this function may also affect the memories we want to keep. Sleep deprivation can also aggravate other menopausal symptoms, such as mood swings and irritability.

One of the most pressing questions women have about menopausal brain fog is whether it is a temporary nuisance or a sign of bigger cognitive challenges ahead. The good news for most women is that it is often temporary, and changes in cognitive performance are typically clinically mild and within normal limits. However, for the remaining women, the impact may be greater.

For most women, brain fog improves as the body adjusts to post-menopausal hormone levels. The worst symptoms typically occur during the perimenopausal phase, when hormone levels fluctuate the most. After menopause, many women find their mental clarity gradually returns.

There is currently no standard assessment for menopausal brain fog. However, psychologists are studying menopausal brain fog to help determine the best therapies. Assessments are being evaluated alongside the need to provide additional information from healthcare professionals, such as fact sheets on how women can best manage brain fog.

It could also be beneficial to check your medications, as some prescriptions and over-the-counter medications may cause side effects that contribute to brain fog.

Some antidepressants, particularly those that affect serotonin levels, opioids, and other pain relievers, can affect cognitive function and contribute to brain fog. In addition, some blood pressure medications can have side effects that impact cognitive clarity.

Antihistamines, often used for allergies, can cause drowsiness and cognitive impairment. While some sleep aids can sometimes lead to grogginess and brain fog.

Taking multiple medications can increase the likelihood of experiencing side effects, such as brain fog. If you suspect that a medication is contributing to your brain fog, it is important to discuss this with your healthcare provider. Always consult a doctor or pharmacist to review potential interactions and alternatives before changing your medications.

If memory loss becomes significant or interferes with your daily activities, it is essential to consult your healthcare provider. Sometimes, these symptoms may signal more serious medical conditions, such as dementia, which require prompt evaluation and care.

It's important to differentiate between temporary lapses in memory, common during menopause and often attributed to brain fog, and the progressive memory loss or confusion characteristic of cognitive decline. Dementia is an umbrella term for conditions that involve a decline in mental functions that disrupt daily life, including difficulties with focus, attention, language skills, problem-solving, and visual perception. Brain fog might explain forgetting a movie title you recently saw, but forgetting you even attended the movie suggests dementia.

Recognizing these distinctions is crucial, but only a healthcare professional can determine the underlying cause of memory concerns. Seeking medical advice allows healthcare professionals to identify potential conditions early, thus ensuring better management and care. Depending on the diagnosis, healthcare providers may recommend a variety of strategies, including lifestyle changes, therapies, or sometimes treatments to address the root cause of your symptoms.

Addressing memory issues can also help provide reassurance and clarity, reducing unnecessary stress or worry. Remember, you don't have to navigate these concerns alone. Your healthcare provider is a valuable resource in understanding and managing your cognitive health. Early discussions and evaluations can empower you to take proactive steps toward maintaining your mental well-being.

3

THE RIPPLE
EFFECTS OF BRAIN FOG

Every year, over 1 million women in the United States experience menopause, marking a significant life transition that brings with it a wide range of physical, emotional, and cognitive changes. Among these changes, menopausal brain fog is a common challenge that manifests uniquely in everyone. For some women, brain fog may present as mild forgetfulness or occasional lapses in concentration, manageable within their daily routines. However, the effects can be far more severe for others, disrupting their ability to focus, think clearly, or remember important information and significantly affecting both personal and professional aspects of life.

This variability in how brain fog affects women underscores the complexity of menopause. Factors such as stress, sleep quality, hormone levels, overall health, and lifestyle contribute to cognitive difficulties experienced. For some women, brain fog may coincide with other symptoms, like fatigue or mood swings, creating a compounded burden that can feel overwhelming.

Despite its prevalence, the challenges of menopausal brain fog are often under-recognized, both socially and within professional environments. This lack of general awareness can leave women feeling unsupported or misunderstood, adding an emotional toll to an already taxing experience. Addressing this requires greater societal education about menopause and its cognitive effects, ensuring women have access to the empathy, resources, and accommodations they need.

Ultimately, by fostering greater understanding and providing tailored support, we can empower women to navigate the complexities of menopause with resilience, confidence, and the knowledge that their experiences are valid and deserving of attention and care. Whether mild or severe, the effects of menopausal brain fog are a reminder of the importance of holistic support for women during this transformative phase of life.

Personal Life Impact

The effect of menopausal brain fog can be devastating for a woman. At home, brain fog can feel like an invisible thief, quietly taking away moments of connection and clarity. Missing birthdays, appointments, or plans with loved ones may cause frustration or hurt feelings. Everyday life turns stressful, with misplaced items, such as your phone left in the fridge or car keys in the pantry, end up becoming part of a routine scavenger hunt. You might even frequently ask, "Did I tell you this already?" as uncertainty creeps into conversations.

Brain fog can leave you feeling emotionally distant or detached, even when you're attempting to stay engaged. You might zone out during conversations, miss important details, or forget to follow up. Your increased irritability or impatience may harm your relationships with loved ones, especially your children, who may be confused by your sudden mood swings, particularly young children. You might doubt your ability to handle responsibilities, both large and small. Embarrassing moments, like forgetting someone's name mid-conversation, can make social interactions feel intimidating.

Finding the right words can feel more like a task than a pleasure, making self-expression difficult. Feeling "not quite yourself" may lead to self-doubt and a sense of inadequacy. These symptoms can disrupt daily routines, creating extra challenges for women juggling family responsibilities and often affecting the entire family dynamic.

To shield yourself from these effects, you might withdraw from relationships and activities you once enjoyed. This withdrawal can lead to women unintentionally creating distance from their partners, causing communication to break down. As a result, partners may feel isolated, and their efforts to help may go unnoticed. When combined with other menopausal symptoms, such as irritability and loss of libido, it's understandable that many partners may experience confusion and a sense of isolation during this time.

However, withdrawing from connections during challenging times can unintentionally intensify the very struggles you aim to manage. Isolation often magnifies the overwhelming emotions and mental fog, creating a cycle where the lack of support exacerbates the brain fog, making it harder to reach out for help. This cycle can leave individuals feeling trapped, compounding their sense of confusion and exhaustion when they most need understanding and encouragement.

For many, the effects of brain fog extend far beyond the individual experiencing it, having a profound impact on relationships within the family. For women, cognitive challenges such as forgetfulness, difficulty concentrating, and reduced mental clarity can lead to frustration and feelings of inadequacy. Family members witnessing these changes may struggle to understand the root cause, which can cause miscommunication, strained relationships, or even feelings of frustration on both sides.

This dynamic can be particularly devastating when it disrupts harmony within a family. Misunderstood symptoms may lead to a sense of disconnection, as women dealing with brain fog feel unable to explain their experiences, and loved ones may feel helpless or uncertain about how to offer support. Over time, this disconnect can erode the emotional bonds within the family, making it even more challenging to cope with the stresses of daily life.

The UK-based Family Law Menopause Project found that 80% of women point to menopause or perimenopause symptoms as impacting their marriage. In the US, adults aged 55 to 64 years have a divorce rate of 46%, with those aged 65 or older showing the greatest increase in the divorce rate between 1990 and 2021. In the UK, women aged 45 to 55 start 40% of all divorce petitions. The Family Law Menopause Project conducted a survey in the UK of law practitioners and found that 81% of family lawyers did not understand or recognize the impact of menopause and perimenopause on divorce and separation. In addition, 65% of all participants that were surveyed agree that women are potentially disadvantaged in terms of financial settlements because of a lack of understanding of "the effect menopause and perimenopause would have on women's earning capability after separation."

Breaking this cycle requires intentional effort to maintain and strengthen connections. Open communication, by sharing your feelings and experiences with loved ones, is key to helping them understand what you're going through and fosters empathy. By encouraging family members to learn about brain fog and its effects, you can create a supportive environment where everyone works together to navigate its challenges.

Leaning on external support systems, such as friends, support groups, or professional counselors, can provide the additional encouragement needed to combat isolation. By actively seeking connection and opening up about your struggles, you can disrupt the cycle of isolation, reduce the weight of brain fog, and foster a sense of shared strength and resilience for both you and your family.

But for some women, unfortunately, while the cognitive challenges of brain fog often improve post-menopause, the lingering effects can persist for years. Symptoms such as lapses in memory, reduced mental clarity, or difficulty concentrating may not immediately disappear, leaving a lasting impact on daily life and professional performance. This can lead to feelings of frustration or self-doubt as women work to rebuild their confidence and adjust to their "new normal."

The emotional and psychological toll of experiencing brain fog during menopause can have long-term effects. During this period, these struggles can negatively affect a woman's overall well-being, including her self-esteem, relationships, and career. The experience of feeling misunderstood or unsupported, especially in work environments, can leave residual feelings of isolation and diminished self-worth.

Addressing these long-term effects begins with fostering understanding and support, both personally and socially. Women can benefit from implementing strategies to improve cognitive health, such as regular exercise, a balanced diet, consistent sleep patterns, and engaging in mentally stimulating activities. Seeking support, whether from friends, family, medical professionals, or support groups, can provide the tools and encouragement needed to manage lingering symptoms effectively.

For society and workplaces, creating awareness about the cognitive challenges associated with menopause is crucial to ensure that women receive the empathy and accommodations they need to thrive. Open conversations, education, and policies that support women through menopause can help reduce the lasting impact of these struggles, empowering them to navigate this phase with resilience and renewed confidence.

Professional Life Impact

In the workplace, menopause brain fog can feel extremely disruptive. After all, this is where sharp thinking, focus, and communication are often non-negotiable. A study conducted by the AARP in 2022 found that some women experience such severe menopausal symptoms it significantly affect those jobs either by causing them to reduce hours or by leaving.

Davina McCall, an English television presenter who is vocal about her menopause experience, is leading the recent push for public discussion on menopause. She has publicly stated that "brain fog" affected her so much that she feared it might be a sign of dementia. It was only when this issue affected her work that she sought help.

Brain fog can manifest in many forms. Multi-tasking, once your superpower, now feels like juggling with one hand tied behind your back. Forgetting deadlines, meeting details, or action items can make you feel unreliable, even if you are working harder than ever. Difficulty focusing or keeping information can slow you down on even routine tasks. Additionally, searching for words or struggling to articulate ideas can shake your confidence in meetings or presentations. You may find yourself pausing longer to find the right phrase, which can lead to worries about how others perceive your competence. Losing track of a thought mid-sentence can also leave you scrambling to recover.

Unfortunately, brain fog often compounds the pressure of high-stakes professional environments. You may spend extra time double-checking your work to avoid mistakes, leading to longer hours and burnout. Fear of being judged or misunderstood can make you hesitant to speak up or take on leadership roles. You may question your abilities and feel out of place in spaces where you once thrived.

The impact is not only on you but may also extend to your colleagues' and or your managers' feelings about you. As a woman approaching her 50s, you may have a successful career and a position of responsibility that reflects the many years of hard work you have put into your career. You are at the top of your field (or almost there), and everything in your career is going well. Everything is under control, and everyone turns to you when something needs doing, as you're the company's key resource. You take on more work and responsibilities, and your team's success stems from your broad knowledge base, allowing you to leverage experiences for efficient workflow. All is well.... until suddenly, it is not.

The lack of communication and awareness surrounding brain fog significantly exacerbates the challenges faced by many women experiencing it. One woman poignantly summarized the struggle: "When things started to slip, instead of talking to me to find out what was wrong, they ignored, sidelined, and abandoned me." This sentiment resonates deeply, reflecting the isolation and frustration that often accompany cognitive difficulties such as brain fog.

Every day, brain fog can affect key cognitive functions like concentration and decision-making, leading to reduced productivity and overall effectiveness in the workplace. Tasks that once felt manageable may seem overwhelming, creating a ripple effect on motivation and enthusiasm for work. This decline in engagement affects individual performance and can also affect workplace dynamics and team productivity.

The long-term consequences of brain fog can sometimes be even more profound. Persistent struggles may cause a decrease in job satisfaction and a growing sense of inadequacy, causing a strain on professional relationships. Misunderstandings or unmet expectations could lead to tensions with colleagues or supervisors, further exacerbating feelings of isolation. Ultimately, these challenges may cause career setbacks, stall professional growth, or even job loss because others often misunderstand or ignore the true nature of the difficulties.

Addressing these issues starts with fostering greater awareness and open dialogue about brain fog. Employers should create environments where employees feel safe discussing cognitive challenges without fear of judgment or stigma. Providing accommodations, such as flexible schedules, regular breaks, or workload adjustments, can go a long way in supporting employees experiencing menopause brain fog. Educational initiatives to inform managers and teams about the symptoms and effects of brain fog can build a culture of understanding and empathy, reducing the likelihood of sidelining those who are struggling.

By acknowledging and addressing the barriers posed by menopause brain fog, we can pave the way for greater inclusivity and support in the workplace. This approach not only benefits those experiencing these challenges but also strengthens teams and organizations, fostering an environment that values and respects all contributions.

Economic Impact

There is currently very little data on the greater economic impact of menopause brain fog, specifically in the U. S., but many women believe menopause hurts their work life. With nearly 20% of the workforce in some phase of menopause, and as high as 60% of women reporting that menopause has negatively affected their work, the impact on the general workforce and the economy is potentially significant.

In a study of 4440 women conducted by The Mayo Clinic, 10% of women reported missing work in the preceding 12 months because of menopause symptoms (median of 3 days missed). This study estimated that these missed workdays could have cost the US $1.8 billion annually. A study with women from the UK, USA, Australia, China, and Japan found that 54% of older women felt they could not discuss issues such as menopause with their employers.

Because brain fog is not an overt physical symptom, people often overlook it as a legitimate cause of decreased workplace performance. As a result, many menopausal women may continue to face challenges in their professional roles, struggling with memory lapses, reduced concentration, or diminished mental clarity. Unfortunately, these struggles often go unrecognized, leaving women at risk of being unfairly judged or dismissed based on perceived declines in productivity.

A quote from an HR manager in the UK sums up the current issues women face: "menopause is a big issue. Thankfully, people are now talking about it, but there's still a real lack of understanding. I've seen where performance is dropping off slightly because of the issues with memory, brain fog, and feeling uncomfortable at work, and it goes down as poor performance. Then, as soon as somebody says, "I'm actually suffering through menopause", it's seen as an excuse. The mindset is not right."

The issues around menopause may also help explain why older women are underrepresented in leadership positions. Studies conducted by Adecco have reported that about 20% of women have lost their jobs because of menopause symptoms, with women in senior positions being the most affected.

This lack of awareness can lead employers to overlook the years of dedication, expertise, and valuable contributions these women have made to their organizations. Instead of acknowledging the physiological changes that may affect performance, some workplaces may unfairly dismiss their struggles as incompetence or a lack of commitment.

In 2022, the UK menopause support app Balance revealed that menopause-related business losses amounted to an alarming £10 billion ($12.15 billion) nationwide. Similarly, research from the Mayo Clinic estimates that menopause costs American companies $26 billion annually, including the $1.8 billion attributed to lost working time alone. On a global scale, Bloomberg reported that menopause-related productivity losses could exceed $150 billion yearly.

Over 1 billion people worldwide will experience menopause by 2025. The once-viable strategy of simply replacing these workers is no longer practical, especially in today's tight labor market and with a shrinking pool of younger workers outside menopause age. Organizations must adapt to keep and support these valuable employees effectively.

To address this issue, it is crucial to foster greater awareness and understanding of the cognitive effects of menopause, including brain fog. Employers should strive to create supportive environments that encourage open dialogue about menopause, implement flexible policies, and provide accommodations to help women navigate this phase. Simple steps, such as offering quiet spaces for focused work or adjusting workloads during particularly challenging periods, can make a meaningful difference. Additionally, education and training for managers and coworkers can help reduce stigma and create a culture of empathy and respect.

A Bank of America study in 2022 determined that companies that embraced gender diversity were more likely to see higher revenues than those that did not. The British Standards Institute suggested that employing 5% more Australians aged 55 or older would boost the national economy by A$48 billion.

On the bright side, companies are slowly making changes. Bristol Myers Squibb received the best-trained workforce award at the 2023 Menopause Friendly Employer Awards, while Microsoft started menopause support for their employees that same year. The award was because of introducing a rounded program for menopause training in the workplace, tailored to address the diverse needs and perspectives of various audience groups.

The UK currently appears to be leading the effort to make businesses more menopause-friendly. In October 2024, the UK government announced that it had appointed journalist and women's rights advocate Mariella Frostrup as the new Menopause Employment Ambassador. In this voluntary role, Mariella will collaborate with employers nationwide to enhance workplace support for women navigating menopause, increase awareness of its symptoms, and highlight the valuable economic contributions of women. A primary focus will assist women experiencing menopause in remaining in the workforce and advancing in their careers.

By acknowledging the challenges of brain fog and implementing workplace policies that promote inclusivity and support, organizations can keep the invaluable skills and experience of menopausal women. Such efforts not only empower these individuals to thrive, but also enrich the workplace with the diverse perspectives and talents that experienced professionals bring. This shift is crucial for fostering equity, so we value and consider everyone's contributions.

4

Understanding Your Brain During Menopause: A Deeper Look

To help understand menopause brain fog, we first need to understand how cognitive function works in the brain. So, what exactly is the cognitive function? Cognitive function refers to the brain's ability to process information, think, learn, remember, and decide.

Brain Structure

An average adult brain weighs about three pounds and contains approximately 60% fat and 40% water, protein, carbohydrates, and salts. While it is not a muscle, the brain is an organ made up of neural tissue. It comprises two distinct types of tissue: gray matter and white matter. Gray matter forms the darker outer layer of the brain, known as the cerebral cortex, and is essential for daily functions such as muscle control, sensory perception, memory, emotional experiences, and speech. White matter lies beneath the gray matter and serves as a communication hub, signaling different parts of the central nervous system to support overall functionality.

The brain divides into three primary regions: the cerebrum, cerebellum, and brainstem. These components work together to power the brain's incredible abilities. The cerebrum regulates and interprets the five senses and conscious actions, such as speech, memory, behavior, personality, movement, reasoning, and judgment. At the back of the brain, near the brainstem, the cerebellum plays a key role in controlling voluntary movements, including balance, posture, coordination, fine motor skills, and speech. The brainstem is critical in regulating automatic body functions that occur without conscious thought, such as heart rate, breathing, sleeping, and swallowing. Positioned at the lower part of the brain, the brainstem serves as a vital connection between the rest of the brain and the spinal cord.

The cerebrum, the brain's largest part, divides into four lobes: frontal, parietal, temporal, and occipital. The frontal lobe, the largest of the lobes, is at the front of the brain, just behind the forehead. It governs essential functions, such as decision-making, problem-solving, consciousness, and emotions. The parietal lobe, at the top of the brain, plays a key role in reacting to information from the body's senses, including touch and temperature, as well as spatial awareness, reading, and interpreting numbers (mathematics). The temporal lobes, positioned on either side of the brain near the ears, handle the understanding of language, learning, memorizing non-verbal information, determining facial expressions, forming words, and remembering verbal information. Meanwhile, the occipital lobe, at the back of the brain, specializes in processing vision, recognizing letters, and distinguishing colors.

The prefrontal cortex, the command center, is in the frontal lobe. In the front part of the brain, the prefrontal cortex manages higher-order thinking skills, such as reasoning, planning, decision-making, impulse control, and problem-solving. It helps regulate attention and working memory, allowing us to hold and manipulate information temporarily. The prefrontal cortex plays a crucial role in goal setting, organization, and adapting to new situations.

The hippocampus, the memory keeper, plays an essential role in memory formation and learning. Located deep within the brain's temporal lobe, the hippocampus converts short-term memories into long-term memories and is essential for learning. Damage to the hippocampus can cause memory loss (as seen in conditions like Alzheimer's disease).

The amygdala, the emotional processor, near the hippocampus, is involved in processing emotions, especially fear and pleasure. It helps encode emotional experiences, making emotionally significant memories stronger. The amygdala also influences decision-making, particularly in situations involving risk or reward.

The basal ganglia, the habit former, is a group of structures deep within the brain that regulate habit formation, motivation, and motor control. They contribute to automatic behaviors, such as driving on familiar routes, and play a role in learning through repetition and reinforcement.

Finally, the thalamus, the information relay, acts as a central hub, relaying sensory information (vision, sound, touch) to different parts of the brain for processing and helps regulate attention, consciousness, and perception, making it vital for cognitive awareness.

Cognitive Function

Cognitive function is crucial for managing daily life and brain activity. It governs thoughts, actions, and how people engage with the world around them. This encompasses the ability to think, learn, and remember, as well as skills such as understanding through thoughts and senses, maintaining attention, learning via memory, decision-making, planning, reasoning, making judgments, speaking, and being aware of one's surroundings. These abilities are central to how we interact with and adapt to our environment.

Two broad categories of cognitive functions exist: perceiving functions and judging functions. Perceiving functions include Sensing and Intuition. Sensing involves processing information from the external world, while Intuition focuses on abstract or conceptual thinking. Judging functions comprise Thinking and Feeling. Thinking relies on logical reasoning and objective analysis for decision-making, whereas Feeling emphasizes personal values and emotions when making choices.

The key aspects of cognitive function are attention, memory, executive function, language processing, problem-solving, reasoning, and perception.

Attention is the ability to focus on specific stimuli while ignoring distractions. This includes selective attention (focusing on one thing), sustained attention (maintaining focus over time), and divided attention (handling multiple tasks at once).

Memory is encoding, storing, and retrieving information. It includes short-term memory (holding small amounts of information temporarily, like a phone number), long-term memory (storing information for extended periods), and working memory (actively manipulating information while using it)

The executive function refers to higher-order processes that involve planning, decision-making, problem-solving, and self-control. The prefrontal cortex plays a significant role in this function.

Language processing is the ability to understand, interpret, and express words and sentences. This involves regions of the cerebrum, such as Broca's area (responsible for speech production), in the left frontal lobe, and Wernicke's area (responsible for language comprehension), in the left temporal lobe.

Problem-solving and reasoning are the ability to analyze situations, draw conclusions, and decide based on logic and experiences.

Perception is the brain's ability to interpret sensory information (sight, sound, touch, etc.) to understand the world.

When performing a cognitive task, multiple brain areas work together in coordination. Reading a book involves the visual cortex (to process words), the language centers (to understand meaning), and the hippocampus (to store information). Solving a problem engages the prefrontal cortex (to analyze information), the basal ganglia (to apply learned strategies), and the cerebellum (to ensure smooth thinking). Experiencing an emotional memory activates the amygdala (to recall emotions) and the hippocampus (to retrieve details).

People once believed that the central nervous system (CNS) solely controlled cognitive function. However, new research reveals that other organ systems and processes also play a role in shaping how we form, process, and store memories, all of which contribute to cognitive function.

5

Cognitive Function: Understanding The Brain's Needs

Cognitive function results from complex interactions between different brain regions, neural networks, nutrients, and external factors. These interactions enable us to think, learn, remember, and process information and involve different parts of the brain interacting to contribute to cognition.

Neurotransmitters

Neurotransmitters (chemical messengers) are chemicals that allow neurons to communicate. When a neuron generates an electrical signal, it triggers the release of neurotransmitters, which cross a small gap between two neurons, called a synapse, to bind with receptors on a neighboring neuron. This process allows the transmission of signals that regulate everything from mood and memory to muscle movement and heart rate. Different neurotransmitters influence cognitive function in various ways. Scientists have identified and categorized at least 100 neurotransmitters based on their chemical properties, including amino acid neurotransmitters.

Amino acid neurotransmitters include glutamate, Gamma-Aminobutyric Acid (GABA), and glycine. Glutamate is the brain's most common excitatory neurotransmitter and plays a key role in cognitive functions like thinking, learning, and memory. While GABA is the brain's most common inhibitory neurotransmitter, it prevents problems in the areas of anxiety, irritability, concentration, sleep, seizures, and depression. Glycine is the most common inhibitory neurotransmitter in your spinal cord and is involved in controlling hearing processing, pain transmission, and metabolism.

Monoamine neurotransmitters regulate consciousness, cognition, attention, and emotion, including serotonin, dopamine, histamine, epinephrine, and norepinephrine.

Serotonin regulates mood, memory, sleep patterns, sexuality, anxiety, appetite, and pain. Dopamine is associated with motivation, focus, concentration, memory, sleep, mood, and motivation. Histamine regulates body functions, including wakefulness, feeding behavior, and motivation. Epinephrine (also called adrenaline) and norepinephrine handle your body's so-called "fight-or-flight response" to fear and stress. Norepinephrine (also called noradrenaline) is most widely known for its effects on alertness, arousal, decision-making, attention, and focus.

While neurotransmitters play a crucial role in communication between neurons, other biological and physiological factors also contribute to brain function and cognition.

Electrical Activity (Neural Firing & Brain Waves)

The brain employs a dual system of communication that involves both neurotransmitters and electrical signals to regulate its intricate functions. Neurons generate action potentials, which are electrical impulses that travel along axons and serve as the primary means of transmitting information. When an action potential reaches the end of a neuron, it triggers the release of neurotransmitters. This coordinated process enables neurons to communicate effectively, playing a crucial role in everything from muscle movement to complex cognitive processes, such as memory and reasoning.

Besides this chemical and electrical interplay, the brain also relies on brainwaves, patterns of electrical activity that reflect different states of consciousness and cognitive functions. These brainwaves operate at various frequencies, each associated with specific mental states: Beta waves link to active thinking and problem-solving, alpha waves to a relaxed but alert state, theta waves to creativity and daydreaming, and delta waves to deep sleep and memory consolidation. This seamless interplay of neurotransmitters, electrical impulses, and brainwave patterns underpins the brain's ability to adapt, process information, and maintain cognitive and emotional health.

Hormones

Unlike neurotransmitters, which act rapidly to transmit signals between neurons, the bloodstream releases hormones, gradually influencing the brain with longer-lasting effects. These chemical messengers play a pivotal role in shaping cognition, emotion, and mental performance.

Key hormones that affect the brain function include cortisol, often referred to as the stress hormone. While low levels of cortisol can help maintain focus and energy, chronic high levels impair memory, concentration, and decision-making, often contributing to mental fatigue. Adrenaline, another stress-related hormone, enhances alertness, boosts reaction speed, and sharpens focus during moments of acute stress, preparing the body and mind for quick action.

Sex hormones such as estrogen and testosterone also have profound effects on brain health. Estrogen supports memory, mood stability, and brain plasticity (the brain's ability to adapt and form new connections). Testosterone, commonly associated with energy and motivation, influences memory and problem-solving skills. Both hormones also contribute to protecting neural structures as we age, highlighting their role in long-term cognitive health.

Thyroid hormones are essential for regulating energy metabolism and maintaining mental clarity. When thyroid hormone levels are imbalanced, individuals often experience symptoms such as brain fog, slower mental processing, or even mood swings. Oxytocin, sometimes called the "bonding hormone," enhances social interactions, emotional intelligence, and trust. It plays a critical role in strengthening interpersonal relationships and building emotional connections.

Together, these hormones act as powerful regulators of brain function, influencing everything from our ability to think critically to the way we connect emotionally with others.

Blood Flow & Oxygen Supply

The brain is also intricately networked with a vast supply of blood vessels, underscoring the vital importance of proper blood flow for optimal cognitive function. The bloodstream serves as the brain's lifeline, delivering oxygen and glucose, essential nutrients that fuel neurons and enable them to function efficiently. These nutrients are critical for sustaining the brain's energy demands, as even a brief disruption in their supply can hinder the ability of neurons to process information, communicate, and regulate various mental and physical functions.

Decreased oxygen availability can lead to sluggish mental processing, memory difficulties, and impaired decision-making. Over time, chronic issues with blood flow may exacerbate the risk of neurodegenerative conditions as the brain becomes more vulnerable to damage from oxidative stress and inflammation.

Stroke, cardiovascular issues, or poor circulation can profoundly reduce blood flow and impact cognitive abilities. Decreased oxygen and glucose availability can lead to sluggish mental processing, memory difficulties, and impaired decision-making. Over time, chronic issues with blood flow may exacerbate the risk of neurodegenerative conditions, as the brain becomes more vulnerable to damage from oxidative stress and inflammation.

Nutrients and Metabolism

Brain function depends on a steady supply of essential nutrients to operate at its best. Glucose is the primary energy source for the brain, fueling its demanding activities and ensuring consistent performance throughout the day. Omega-3 fatty acids, found in foods like fatty fish and walnuts, play a crucial role in maintaining the structure of neurons and enhancing communication between brain cells, which is vital for effective cognitive functioning and memory.

Besides these macronutrients, specific vitamins are essential for brain health. Vitamin B12 supports the formation of red blood cells and helps maintain the myelin sheath, a protective layer around neurons that ensures the efficient transmission of signals. Vitamin D plays a multifaceted role, contributing to neural function and reducing the risk of neurodegenerative diseases. Meanwhile, vitamin E acts as a powerful antioxidant, protecting brain cells from oxidative stress, which can lead to cognitive decline.

Antioxidants found in fruits and vegetables combat oxidative stress, safeguarding brain cells from damage.

Brain Rewiring

Neuroplasticity is the brain's ability to reorganize and rewire itself in response to learning, experiences, and environmental changes. This adaptability is a cornerstone of cognitive development, allowing the brain to strengthen or create new neural connections. The strength and number of synaptic connections, the points where neurons communicate, are critical for determining how efficiently we think, learn, and remember. With each repeated experience, the brain reinforces specific neural pathways, making certain skills or behaviors more automatic and deeply ingrained.

This process is why practice and repetition play such an essential role in skill acquisition. Mastering a musical instrument or tackling complex problem-solving tasks can stimulate the brain's plasticity, promoting the growth of new connections and strengthening existing ones. Over time, these efforts make tasks that once felt challenging become second nature.

Neuroplasticity is not only important for learning, but also for recovery. Following an injury, such as a stroke, the brain can adapt by rerouting functions through alternate neural pathways, enabling individuals to regain lost abilities.

Besides recovering from injuries, neuroplasticity allows us to adjust to changing circumstances throughout life. For example, moving to a new environment or adapting to a new job can stimulate the brain's ability to reorganize and learn, ensuring that we remain capable and adaptive in the face of change.

External Factors

External factors can influence brain function, as the brain constantly processes information from sight, sound, touch, smell, and taste. Learning and mental stimulation—through activities like problem-solving, reading, or playing an instrument—reinforce neural pathways and enhances cognitive abilities. Physical activity increases blood flow, promotes neurogenesis (the creation of new neurons), and supports memory improvement. Sleep plays a crucial role, with deep sleep helping in memory consolidation and the removal of brain toxins. Lastly, stress and trauma can negatively affect neurons, particularly in the hippocampus, which is essential for memory and learning.

Cognitive function is a complex and dynamic process that engages various brain structures, neural pathways, and neurotransmitters. It enables the brain to integrate sensory input, emotions, experiences, and knowledge, allowing us to navigate life effectively. Cognitive abilities often evolve with age, though memory and processing speed may sometimes decline. Lifestyle factors strongly influence brain health, such as diet, exercise, sleep, and mental engagement. Additionally, stress, anxiety, and depression can play a significant role in affecting cognitive function.

The term "brain fog" describes a range of symptoms that disrupt cognitive function, hindering clear thinking, focus, concentration, memory, and attention. As the name suggests, these symptoms create a sense of mental cloudiness, making everyday tasks like holding conversations, following instructions, or recalling steps more difficult to handle.

Frequent symptoms of brain fog during menopause include memory and attention problems, difficulty keeping and recalling language, distractibility, difficulty concentrating, forgetting intentions (such as why one entered a room), and problems switching tasks.

6

Hormones And Brain Fog: The Missing Link?

Menopause is a natural process that shows the end of a woman's reproductive age and occurs when a woman enters her 40s or 50s. Currently, the average age for menopause is 52 years in the United States. The official diagnosis for menopause is the point when 12 months have passed without a menstrual period.

Perimenopause is the period before menopause, whereby a woman may have menopause-like symptoms like irregular periods, hot flashes, and more but is still menstruating. Perimenopause, on average, lasts about 4 years. However, this can occur up to 10 years before menopause.

Post-menopause is the period after menopause and lasts for the rest of your life. It is also the time when the common menopausal symptoms will most likely stop. However, while most women find that the majority, if not all, of their symptoms of menopause, ease up in post-menopause, some women continue to experience symptoms for several years or longer in the post-menopause period.

Estrogen

The end of your monthly period occurs because of your ovaries' reduced estrogen production. Estrogen, a hormone produced by the ovaries between puberty and menopause, regulates periods and helps prepare the uterus for a potential pregnancy each month. While often thought of as a "female hormone," estrogen's influence extends far beyond reproductive health as it also helps with blood pressure, heart health, bone density, muscle mass, and brain health.

Researchers have established for some time that estrogen is neuroprotective, meaning it helps protect nerve endings. As a result, estrogen may help safeguard the hippocampus from damage, which could protect against brain fog and cognitive decline. In addition, there are several other ways estrogen might affect the hippocampus, the part of the brain that plays a significant role in memory formation, spatial navigation, and emotional regulation.

Researchers are still investigating the effects of estrogen on the brain and hippocampus. However, they have discovered that estrogen may help increase the number of spines in the brain. These spines branch off nerve cells and are essential for brain cell communication. Therefore, estrogen may enhance communication between brain cells in the hippocampus, potentially assisting with memory.

While evidence shows that estrogen positively affects learning, memory, and mood, many believe low estrogen levels cause concentration difficulties and mood swings. Estrogen receptors, cellular proteins that bind estrogen to induce a response, are present throughout the brain, particularly in areas that regulate temperature and the sleep-wake cycle. Decreasing estrogen levels results in less interaction with the receptors, reducing the estrogen response. Brain fog may then occur when estrogen cannot activate the memory center of the brain.

Results from a small study using Positron Emission Tomography (PET) scans to look at the brains of 54 healthy premenopausal, perimenopausal, and postmenopausal women found that the number of estrogen receptors in the brain increases as a woman goes through menopause. This increase in estrogen receptors persisted for up to 15 years after menopause and correlated with a decline in cognitive function like brain fog. Further research is required, but scientists think the brain may increase the number of estrogen receptors to compensate for the lower estrogen levels. Maintaining estrogen levels may therefore help delay the increase in the number of estrogen receptors in the brain.

In addition, low estrogen levels affect brain function by contributing to lower levels of serotonin and dopamine (neurotransmitters), making you feel forgetful and less mentally sharp, which are both symptoms of menopausal brain fog. Studies have shown that in women experiencing menopausal hot flashes, restricted blood flow to the brain potentially affects the brain's needed oxygen and nutrients.

Low levels of estrogen may also contribute to sleep problems, as well as depression and anxiety. Sleep disruption at any age has the potential to affect memory and attention, so when combined with low estrogen-induced hot flashes during menopause, this may also add to challenges for the brain. Insomnia affects between 35-65% of menopausal or perimenopausal women, and studies have shown that estrogen therapy reduces insomnia.

Therefore, during menopause, when estrogen levels decline, besides the physical symptoms of menopause, the reduction in the positive effects on the brain systems might cause it to slow down, causing the symptoms of brain fog: forgetfulness, trouble concentrating, and mental fatigue.

While estrogen is the primary focus during menopause, other hormonal changes may also contribute to brain fog during menopause.

Progesterone

Progesterone is a hormone whose primary function during a woman's fertile years is to prepare the uterus to accept and carry a fertilized egg. By preventing muscle contractions in the uterus, progesterone stops a woman's body from rejecting a fertilized egg. Like estrogen, as a woman approaches menopause, the body makes less progesterone.

Progesterone's crucial role in many vital brain functions, besides its effects on the reproductive cycle, makes it a neurosteroid. Several clinical research studies have shown that progesterone may have protective qualities in the brain, a characteristic known as "neuroprotection," with studies showing a link between progesterone and improved cognitive function.

Besides promoting healthy brain function, scientists believe that progesterone protects the brain from damage and helps repair it after injury. They believe progesterone does this by repairing the myelin sheath and promoting neurogenesis.

Studies have also shown that progesterone has a sleep-promoting effect. As a result, low levels of progesterone can contribute to sleep issues such as reduced ability to fall and stay asleep or to experience a deep restorative sleep.

During perimenopause, your estrogen and progesterone levels are on a wild rollercoaster ride, which gradually slows down as you approach menopause itself. Progesterone is the first hormone to decline during menopause, and its reduced levels can lead to sleep disruptions, mood swings, irritability, and brain fog.

Testosterone

The ovaries and adrenal glands release testosterone into the bloodstream of women at levels approximately 10 to 20 times lower than in men. Testosterone plays a role in bone health, regulates other hormones, and is involved in reproductive health and libido. It also contributes to mental sharpness and clarity by strengthening the nerves.

Like estrogen and progesterone, testosterone also declines as women age, and at the time of menopause, it is, on average, a quarter of what the level was at its highest. However, currently, there is no level at which testosterone is classified as being low, and proper levels will depend on the individual woman.

Testosterone also acts on the arteries that supply blood to the brain. Thus, it helps to prevent memory loss, as well as helps to maintain mental sharpness and clarity by supporting the nerves in the brain. While clinical studies have shown that testosterone significantly influences cognitive function, mood regulation, and social behavior, no controlled clinical studies in menopausal women have shown that testosterone is beneficial in helping with brain fog.

In their 2019 global consensus position statement on the use of testosterone therapy for women, the International Menopause Society stated that there is currently insufficient evidence to support the use of testosterone to enhance cognitive performance or delay cognitive decline in postmenopausal women.

Thyroid Hormone

Brain fog is also a symptom of hypothyroidism. Therefore, women around menopause often receive diagnoses of thyroid hormone issues because of similar symptoms.

The thyroid gland produces thyroid hormones, primarily comprising two hormones: thyroxine (T4) and triiodothyronine (T3). Together, these hormones regulate the body's metabolism. Hypothyroidism occurs when the thyroid gland becomes underactive and cannot produce enough thyroid hormone. Low levels of thyroid hormones are associated with fatigue, forgetfulness, and difficulty concentrating.

Levothyroxine, a synthetic form of thyroid hormone thyroxine, is a common treatment for hypothyroidism. A clinical study examining the effects of levothyroxine during menopause in hypothyroid women suggested that cognitive function in hypothyroid women taking levothyroxine during menopause is comparable to that of women who are not hypothyroid. The study also noted that hypothyroid women taking levothyroxine showed slightly better processing speed and working memory compared to women without hypothyroidism.

There have, however, been no studies with levothyroxine in menopausal brain fog. Because unnecessary levothyroxine use can cause adverse effects, speak with a healthcare provider before use.

Cortisol

Cortisol, a stress hormone produced by the adrenal glands, plays a vital role in regulating the body's stress response. Beyond stress management, cortisol also supports other essential functions, such as maintaining metabolism, regulating blood pressure, and helping the body transition from sleep to wakefulness.

Research shows that cortisol levels rise in some women as they approach menopause. Elevated cortisol can suppress estrogen production, which may influence cognitive function, including memory performance. This disruption may contribute to symptoms of brain fog, such as difficulty concentrating or remembering information.

More frequent and intense hot flashes in women are associated with increased stress, a known trigger of cortisol release. This can create a harmful cycle where the physical and emotional toll of stress amplifies cortisol production, exacerbating symptoms and making it harder to break free from the cycle.

Effects of Hormonal Changes

While hormones naturally change during menopause, the hormonal shifts experienced during menopause can increase risks for certain conditions that also affect brain health, such as cardiovascular disease or diabetes.

Research shows that estrogen protects the heart by increasing blood flow, preventing free radical damage to arteries, and raising good cholesterol (HDL) while lowering bad cholesterol (LDL). Studies also show that women experiencing menopause in their 40s face more cardiovascular problems than those who experience it later. Cardiovascular diseases may then affect brain function, with the impact dependent on the type of cardiovascular disease. For example, studies report a 39% increased risk of memory or thinking problems in atrial fibrillation patients.

Hormones also affect the body's insulin response. As estrogen and progesterone levels change after menopause, blood sugar levels may fluctuate more than they did before menopause. The human brain uses about half of all the energy produced by sugar. If sugar levels drop below normal, it can damage the nerves in the brain, leading to memory and learning issues. Consequently, women with diabetes may need to monitor their blood sugar levels more frequently during menopause.

7

HRT: Help Or Hindrance?

Hormone replacement therapy (HRT) can be a valuable option for many women experiencing menopause. It helps address symptoms like hot flashes, mood swings, and low libido and supports bone health by replacing declining hormones, such as estrogen, progesterone, and testosterone. Healthcare providers determine the type and dose of hormones based on individual needs and their recommendations. Healthcare providers typically start HRT at the lowest dose and adjust it as needed. While it's commonly used for 2 to 5 years, the duration can vary based on each woman's unique circumstances.

HRT is available in a variety of forms, including pills, patches, and gels, which can contain individual hormones or a combination. Pills are a traditional and simpler option, though they may cause digestive side effects and carry a higher risk of blood clots. Patches and gels offer a steady hormone release, and women who wish to avoid daily pills often prefer them. Low-dose estrogen comes in options like creams, gels, vaginal tablets, pessaries, or rings that are inserted into the vagina. These are helpful for managing menopausal symptoms, such as vaginal dryness, burning sensations, or discomfort during sex.

The type of HRT you need may depend on whether you've had a hysterectomy. If you still have your womb, you'll usually need both estrogen and progestogen. Progestogens help reduce the risk of womb cancer by preventing excessive growth of the uterine lining growth, reducing the risk of endometrial cancer.

Some researchers suggest that if estrogen influences the hippocampus and other brain regions, hormone replacement therapy (HRT) might help ease brain fog. This may be because estrogen interacts with brain receptors. Estrogen may ease symptoms of brain fog linked to fatigue or mood changes. For example, HRT can ease night sweats, improving sleep and reducing foggy, tired thinking.

A study of 693 postmenopausal women, with an average age of 52.6 years and 1.4 years post-menopause, showed that oral HRT did not improve cognitive function. However, transdermal estrogen showed a small to moderate positive effect on mood for up to four years, with no data available beyond that timeframe. Another study involving 567 women found that starting estradiol within six years of menopause did not significantly affect verbal memory, executive function, or overall cognition compared to therapy started over ten years after menopause.

A larger study of 1,326 postmenopausal women, who took part in two randomized placebo-controlled trials over an average of seven years (ages 50–55), found that conjugated equine estrogen (CEE)-based therapies neither offered sustained cognitive benefits nor posed risks for cognitive function. The data does not address whether starting and continuing HRT during menopause until symptoms subside affects cognitive function in the short or long term. Notably, these studies primarily examined oral estrogen and not the transdermal forms (gels and patches) now available.

Although smaller studies and case reports suggest testosterone might improve brain fog, a larger meta-analysis found no consistent evidence to support its benefits. Currently, no consensus exists to confirm that testosterone significantly affects thinking or memory.

At this time, the effectiveness of HRT in easing menopausal brain fog remains uncertain. The Food and Drug Administration in the United States has, to date, only approved HRT to treat some physical symptoms of menopause in postmenopausal women. There are currently no approved drugs in the United States to treat brain fog for menopausal women. Researchers haven't thoroughly studied HRT's impact on peri- or menopausal women, but treating other menopausal symptoms may ease brain fog.

You should consult a healthcare provider to determine if HRT is appropriate for you based on your medical history and risk factors before beginning any treatment. Healthcare providers should discuss both the risks and benefits of HRT with you, as all FDA-approved estradiol drugs carry significant warnings and may not be suitable for all women.

As you age, especially after 60, the risks of HRT may outweigh its benefits. Menopause symptoms often ease over time, reducing the need for HRT. However, prolonged use of combined HRT can increase the risk of breast cancer. For those who wish to start or continue HRT after 60, a healthcare provider might recommend a low dose and suggest using patches or gels instead of tablets to help minimize risks.

It's important that you become an effective self-advocate about your health by having in-depth conversations with your healthcare provider about your overall health and any symptoms, whether or not, prompted. Remember to discuss all your symptoms with your healthcare provider, as there may be other potential contributing factors to your brain fog that are not menopause related. This ensures that you address all potential underlying medical conditions.

8

Fueling Mental Clarity

Can diet help menopause brain fog? When menopause, brain fog, sets in, it is easy to feel like clarity is out of reach. Reducing stress, managing time, and maintaining good health may help. Practical lifestyle changes might transform menopause brain fog from an overwhelming problem into a manageable challenge.

The foods you eat can have a direct impact on your brain function. As menopause can increase inflammation, which then affects brain health, eating plenty of fruits and vegetables, which are rich in antioxidants, may counter this effect. Consuming healthy fats can also support brain function while eating protein helps stabilize blood sugar, which prevents energy dips and mental sluggishness.

A Mediterranean diet may be beneficial to brain health in postmenopausal women as it is rich in fruits, vegetables, whole grains, and healthy fats, and is rich in plant estrogens (e.g., flaxseeds, sesame seeds, and beans).

Soy contains a high concentration of isoflavones, which are plant-based compounds that have similar, albeit weaker, effects to estrogen. Besides isoflavones, soy also provides B vitamins, fiber, potassium, magnesium, and protein. The estrogen-like action of soy isoflavones has led to their promotion as beneficial for alleviating menopausal symptoms.

A review of 16 randomized controlled studies involving 1386 adults with a mean age of 60 years found that eating soy isoflavones improved overall cognitive function and memory in adults. Researchers only observed improved visual memory (memory for faces) in a 2.5-year study of 350 postmenopausal women aged 45-92 years. In a review conducted by The Menopause Society (formerly known as the North American Menopause Society), the effects of soy-based isoflavones had mixed results. However, early findings potentially showed the benefits of isoflavone more on cognitive function in younger postmenopausal women than in older women. There are potential downsides, however, to eating soy, as it can interact with many medications that can affect thyroid function in people with iodine deficiency and might lower immune responses and cause cancer.

Other food items beneficial to the brain include proteins, omega-3 fatty acids, and vitamins such as B and D. Proteins from meats, poultry, dairy, cheese, and eggs contain amino acids, which are the building blocks of protein. These amino acids also play a role in metabolism, cell signaling, and the production of hormones and neurotransmitters. Consuming sufficient protein can boost your mood, mental health, and work performance. Researchers at Harvard studied 77,000 men and women over 20 years and found that for every 5% of calories from plant protein instead of carbohydrates, the risk of developing dementia decreased by 26%, compared to an 11% decrease when animal protein replaced carbohydrates. For every additional three servings of peas and lima beans consumed weekly, there was a 28% lower risk of cognitive decline. Beans and legumes were determined to be the most protective against cognitive decline. However, animal protein provides all nine essential amino acids that the body cannot produce on its own, which are important for other functions such as muscle growth and immune health.

Omega-3 Fatty Acids

Omega-3 fatty acids can support brain health and help ease certain symptoms of brain fog, such as difficulties with attention and memory. These beneficial fats appear in salmon, mackerel, tuna, sardines, and fish oil. Fish oil contains two key types of omega-3 fatty acids: eicosapentaenoic acid (EPA) and docosahexaenoic acid (DHA). Studies show DHA, the brain's primary omega-3 fatty acid, influences neurotransmitters and enhances brain function. A review of nine studies involving 1,319 adults, 55.19% of whom were women, revealed that consuming omega-3 fatty acids improves learning, memory, and cognitive health while also boosting blood flow in the brain.

Vitamins

You can find vitamin B, an essential nutrient for brain wellness, in eggs, whole grains, fish, avocados, and citrus fruits. Studies show that B vitamins play a vital role in mood and cognitive function. Low levels of B12, B6, and folate are linked to two common brain fog symptoms: memory problems and difficulty concentrating.

Vitamin C, often associated with immune health, has also been linked to brain fog. Low levels of vitamin C impair memory, attention, and focus, and may contribute to depression and cognitive impairment. In one study, researchers found that vitamin C supplementation improved memory and attention performance. Oranges, strawberries, kiwis, broccoli, and red bell peppers all contain vitamin C.

Studies have linked low levels of Vitamin D to brain fog symptoms such as poor concentration and memory problems. Vitamin D also stabilizes mood and is present in dairy products, beef liver, orange juice, and egg yolks. Sun exposure generates vitamin D in the skin; however, excessive sun exposure increases the risk of skin cancer.

Vitamin E is a powerful antioxidant that helps safeguard cells from damage caused by oxidative stress from free radicals. It is abundant in foods such as sunflower seeds, almonds, spinach, avocados, squash, kiwifruit, trout, shrimp (prawns), olive oil, wheat germ oil, and broccoli. However, a 2021 study found no definitive evidence to support vitamin E's effectiveness in improving mild cognitive impairment.

Minerals

Iron is a vital mineral essential for producing blood, transporting oxygen, and supporting overall growth and development. Various sources, including meat, seafood, fortified foods, grains, and nuts, provide iron. Research suggests that imbalances in iron levels, whether too high or too low, may affect nervous system function, potentially leading to changes in memory, attention, and behavior, all of which are linked to brain fog.

Studies show that magnesium supports brain health, and low levels are associated with brain fog. Besides alleviating brain fog, magnesium also improves cognitive function and reduces susceptibility to stress. Leafy green vegetables, nuts, seeds, and whole grains are all rich in magnesium.

Zinc plays an essential role in maintaining brain health and cognitive function. It is critical for brain signaling and helping neurons communicate effectively, which supports memory and learning. Zinc also has anti-inflammatory properties, reducing inflammation in the brain that can negatively affect mental clarity. This makes it a vital nutrient for both maintaining focus and protecting against cognitive decline.

Copper is integral to the production of neurotransmitters, the chemical messengers that neurons use to communicate. This mineral facilitates the transmission of signals between brain cells, ensuring seamless communication that is vital for memory, focus, and emotional regulation. Copper also supports the overall health of neural structures, playing a significant role in maintaining cognitive performance.

Iodine, a key element for thyroid health, indirectly supports brain function by regulating metabolism and energy levels. The thyroid hormones it helps produce are essential for proper brain development and function. When iodine levels are adequate, the brain benefits from stable energy production, which is critical for maintaining mental clarity, focus, and efficient cognitive processes.

Calcium is essential for neurotransmitter release and neural communication. Calcium supports cognitive processes like memory and focus. Low calcium levels can disrupt these functions, potentially leading to mental fatigue and brain fog.

Choline is a precursor to acetylcholine, a neurotransmitter critical for memory and learning. Choline helps maintain mental clarity. Insufficient choline can impair cognitive function, contributing to symptoms of brain fog.

Manganese supports enzyme activity in the brain and protects against oxidative stress. A deficiency in manganese may hinder neural connectivity and cognitive performance, exacerbating brain fog.

Chromium, by regulating glucose metabolism, ensures a steady energy supply to the brain. Fluctuations in blood sugar levels, often linked to low chromium, can cause mental fatigue and fogginess.

Molybdenum, while not directly linked to cognition, supports metabolic processes that are essential for maintaining overall brain health. Deficiencies in molybdenum may indirectly affect mental clarity.

Potassium is vital for maintaining neural communication and electrical activity in the brain. Potassium imbalances can disrupt focus, memory, and overall cognitive function, contributing to brain fog.

Incorporating these essential minerals into your diet through nutrient-rich foods like seafood, nuts, seeds, whole grains, and leafy greens can help maintain optimal brain health. If you suspect deficiencies, consult a healthcare professional for guidance on supplementation to ensure your brain thrives.

While vitamins, minerals, and supplements can support cognitive function, it's important to approach them with caution. Taking excessive amounts can lead to harmful side effects, interact with medications, or disrupt your body's natural balance. Always consult a healthcare professional before starting any supplement regimen to ensure it's safe and tailored to your needs.

Water

Dehydration occurs when your body lacks the necessary fluids. This can result from not drinking enough water, excessive fluid loss through sweating or urination, or a condition that reduces your body's ability to retain fluids. Staying properly hydrated is essential, and a good guideline is to drink enough water to ensure your urine is light yellow or clear. If you're exercising, it's especially important to increase your water intake to replace the fluids lost through sweat. Monitoring the color of your urine can help you check your hydration levels, as dark yellow usually indicates dehydration.

Dehydration can exacerbate brain fog, so women need to stay hydrated by drinking water regularly throughout the day. Water plays a vital role in supporting various brain functions. Studies have found that even mild dehydration (1-2% of body weight) can lead to reduced concentration, mood swings, and increased difficulty in completing tasks. Dehydration also reduces blood volume, thus delivering less oxygen and nutrients to the brain.

Staying hydrated is especially important if you experience menopause symptoms like hot flashes and night sweats, as sweating can lead to increased fluid loss. Drinking eight glasses of water a day may not be enough, particularly if you live in a hot and humid climate or engage in physical activity that causes you to sweat more than usual.

While dehydration can contribute to brain fog, certain drinks can make it worse. Caffeinated beverages, for example, act as diuretics, causing you to lose more fluids than you take in, which can exacerbate dehydration. Alcohol is also a diuretic and can further dehydrate your body. Sugary drinks may worsen dehydration as well, as they speed up fluid loss and can lead to brain fog through sugar crashes. To manage dehydration and brain fog effectively, avoiding these beverages and prioritizing water intake is essential.

Alcohol Reduction

Drinking alcohol during menopause can often exacerbate the symptoms of menopause and increase the risk of other health conditions. As women age, they are less likely to burn off the calories from alcohol, thus making it more difficult to keep their weight at a healthy level. Carrying extra weight may then increase the risk of other diseases. In addition, as women age, they have less of the enzyme, alcohol dehydrogenase, which metabolizes alcohol in the stomach, which increases the amount of alcohol absorbed into the blood.

Moderate alcohol consumption (one drink per day) may increase estrogen levels in women receiving HRT, while alcohol did not affect hormone levels in women not receiving it. However, there are conflicting data on the benefits of alcohol during menopause. One survey found that women who drank alcohol daily were more likely to report hot flashes and night sweats. While another study found that light, infrequent alcohol consumption may help relieve hot flashes.

Results from a UK study have suggested that moderate (1 drink per day) alcohol consumption may help decrease a menopausal woman's risk for heart disease. A South Korean study determined that moderate alcohol consumption may significantly boost bone density. In addition, moderate drinking is also associated with a lower risk of type 2 diabetes, dementia, and obesity.

However, excess alcohol consumption during menopause is associated with an increased risk of conditions such as cancer, heart problems, liver disease, and osteoporosis.

Alcohol can also affect the quality of sleep by disrupting the sleep cycle and causing dehydration, which compounds the sleep difficulties many menopausal women already face, leading to further exhaustion and a decline in overall well-being. Additionally, alcohol can exacerbate mood changes, depression, heightened anxiety, and irritability because of hormonal adjustments, affecting mood regulation. This can lead to an intensification of these feelings over time. For women already experiencing mental health challenges during menopause, alcohol can make managing emotions even more difficult.

9

Balancing Mind And Body For Mental Clarity

Balancing the mind and body may help combat brain fog and reclaim mental clarity. By nurturing both physical health and mental well-being, women can create a harmonious foundation for optimal cognitive function. The following are practical strategies and lifestyle adjustments that may help counter the effects of menopause brain fog.

The multi-racial and multi-ethnic SWAN study revealed that financial hardship and hypertension, frequently associated with stress, are major factors in cognitive decline.

Sleep Improvement Habits

Menopause causes frequent disruptions of sleep patterns because of the intimate connection between sleep and brain health. Because of this intimate connection, restless nights may leave your brain struggling to recharge from the stress and anxiety of worrying about your menopause symptoms, potentially leading to insomnia. Without good sleep, even the best habits will not fully combat brain fog, so sleep is your brain's chance to reset, recharge, and clear away mental clutter.

While sleep deprivation affects how clearly you think and interferes with your memory and learning abilities, it may also reduce your attention span and slow your brain. You may also find that you get decision fatigue, and sometimes you may find you have stronger reactions to stressful situations, such as in the workplace, as your brain finds it more difficult to see the positive side of things.

Ample sleep works to restore these effects by actively refining the brain's ability to make new connections. To encourage sufficient sleep, it's helpful to calm the brain before bed. Activities such as reading, gentle stretching, or meditation can be beneficial. It is best to limit any screen time before bed, as the blue light from electronic devices can interfere with your body's natural sleep-wake cycle, thus disrupting your sleep.

To promote better sleep, your bedroom should be dark, quiet, and cool. Given the time we spend sleeping and the importance of sleep for the body, it is worthwhile to invest in a comfortable mattress and pillows.

Stress Reduction Techniques

The demands of modern life often require juggling multiple roles, work, family, and personal responsibilities. As a result, many women routinely feel stressed, which can then contribute to and amplify the effects of menopause brain fog.

Hormonal changes, particularly fluctuations in estrogen and progesterone levels, which can affect cognitive function, often cause menopause brain fog. Stress can exacerbate these cognitive difficulties by increasing anxiety, disrupting sleep, and affecting overall cognitive function. Stress management can, therefore, help regulate hormone levels.

One technique to help manage stress is meditation. Studies show that regular meditation lowers cortisol levels, thus reducing stress-related cognitive impairments. One small study on slow-paced breathing involving 34 middle-aged women showed an improvement in cognitive performance among postmenopausal women.

Other techniques include taking regular exercise, eating a healthy diet, and getting adequate sleep. Regular exercise, such as walking, running, yoga, or dancing, can lead to the release of endorphins, which helps reduce stress. A healthy diet supports your overall health and stress resilience, while adequate sleep ensures you get enough restful rest to recharge your body and mind.

Overall, managing your stress levels through relaxation techniques, regular exercise, and a healthy lifestyle can help mitigate the effects of menopausal brain fog.

Exercise

Clinical trials show that regular exercise improves the health of postmenopausal women, and researchers have found a link between long-term physical exercise and reduced rates of cognitive decline.

Women who did aerobics 3x a week for 12 weeks reported improvements in sleep quality, insomnia, and depression in late perimenopausal or postmenopausal sedentary women compared to women who did not take part in the exercise program. The increase in blood flow to the brain caused by brisk exercise may also help brain fog.

Studies have also shown that less intense exercise is beneficial. Although researchers didn't study data specific to the benefits related to brain fog, therapeutic walking programs for menopausal women (ranging from 4 weeks to 3 years) demonstrated benefits. 91% of walking programs studied showed a beneficial outcome in at least one menopause-related medical issue.

Strength training helps regulate hormones and stabilizes mood. It is especially important during menopause to maintain muscle mass and bone health. Stretch or do light yoga to reduce tension and increase blood flow to your brain.

Mental Exercise

Stimulating the brain through cognitive exercises can help you navigate brain fog. The brain loves novelty, as it helps stimulate it. Memory games such as list recall challenges, match up games, and storytelling can all help stimulate focus and concentration by stimulating the parts of the brain responsible for memory and recall. Even learning a new language can help manage brain fog by stimulating your brain.

Crossword puzzles, Sudoku, jigsaws, and brain teasers help mitigate the effects of brain fog by stimulating the brain. While crossword puzzles enhance memory recall, jigsaw puzzles improve concentration.

Sudoku enhances problem-solving skills, and brain teasers aid cognitive flexibility.

Social interactions also play a crucial role in mitigating cognitive decline, making it important to maintain your social connections. People who regularly gather with friends and family, volunteer, or attend classes tend to have more robust gray matter and healthier brains. To enhance your brain's gray matter and overall well-being, avoid social isolation and cultivate safe social interactions.

Digital Overload

The modern world often inundates the brain with distractions and stressors, exacerbating the symptoms of brain fog. Today's constant connectivity and "always-on" culture create mental overload; endless notifications and social media interruptions demand attention, hindering focus and effective information processing. These frequent interruptions can interfere with memory formation and concentration, leaving your mind feeling fragmented and overwhelmed.

Balancing many responsibilities with insufficient downtime can further hinder your brain's ability to process and organize information. Rapid task-switching, often required in a fast-paced lifestyle, taxes cognitive resources, reducing your capacity for deep, focused thinking. Spending prolonged hours online can amplify this effect, contributing to mental fatigue and diminishing your ability to fully engage in meaningful activities.

To counteract these challenges, consider adopting a digital detox to restore mental clarity. Stepping away from devices, even for short periods, can help reduce mental clutter, allowing your mind to recharge and refocus. Use this time to reconnect with offline activities, such as reading a book, spending time outdoors, engaging in creative hobbies, or simply enjoying moments of stillness. Incorporating regular breaks from technology into your routine can lead to improved cognitive function, better attention span, and a stronger sense of mental balance.

By deliberately creating space for rest and reconnection, you can empower your brain to recover from the demands of modern life, fostering a clearer, more focused mind and enhancing your overall well-being.

10

Navigating The Emotional Journey Of Brain Fog

Menopausal brain fog can introduce emotional challenges such as frustration, self-doubt, and anxiety, as concentrating and recalling information become more difficult. These changes may feel unsettling, affecting confidence and daily interactions. Recognizing that these emotions may stem from natural hormonal fluctuations can help ease their impact. By acknowledging and addressing these feelings with empathy and care, individuals can navigate this phase with improved clarity and emotional strength.

Self-Compassion

Derived from Latin, the term "self-compassion" reflects the idea of being "with suffering" (com = with, passion = suffering). It represents a positive and empathetic attitude we can adopt toward ourselves and is also a measurable concept in psychology. Introduced into positive psychology by Associate Professor Dr. Kristin Neff, self-compassion comprises three core elements: self-kindness, common humanity, and mindfulness.

Self-compassion involves turning inward and offering yourself the same understanding and kindness you'd naturally extend to a friend in times of struggle or self-doubt. It means being supportive when facing challenges, feelings of inadequacy, or mistakes. Instead of ignoring pain with a "stiff upper lip" approach or becoming overwhelmed by negative thoughts and emotions, self-compassion encourages you to pause and ask, "This is difficult. How can I care for and comfort myself right now?"

Self-kindness involves recognizing your inherent worth, even when you fall short of your expectations. To practice self-compassion, treat yourself as you would a close friend, allow room for mistakes, and offer yourself the same care and understanding you extend to others. Sometimes, it's as simple as acknowledging your feelings and resisting the urge to be overly critical of yourself.

Building Emotional Resilience

Emotional resilience is the ability to calm your mind after facing a negative experience and effectively handle and recover from life's challenges. It can make the difference between maintaining composure under pressure and feeling overwhelmed. Resilient individuals adopt a more positive outlook and manage stress more efficiently.

Research suggests that while some people may naturally possess resilience, it is possible to cultivate these behaviors. Building resilience often starts with believing in yourself and having confidence in your ability to navigate life's stresses. Positive thinking, however, doesn't mean ignoring your problems; instead, it involves recognizing that setbacks are temporary and that you have the skills to overcome them.

Nurturing yourself is essential. During stressful times, it's common to neglect self-care, such as eating well, exercising, or getting enough sleep. To strengthen resilience, focus on self-care even when life feels overwhelming. Make time for activities that bring you joy and help you recharge.

Journaling

According to Amy Hoyt, PhD, founder of Mending Trauma, "Journaling can serve as a great pressure-releasing valve when we feel overwhelmed or simply have a lot going on internally."

A 2019 study involving patients, families, and healthcare practitioners from a children's hospital found that journaling exercises led to reduced stress levels. Researchers asked participants to write three things they were grateful for, create a six-word story of their life, and list three personal wishes. In a follow-up 12 to 18 months later, 85% of participants found the exercise helpful, and 59% continued journaling to manage stress.

A 2018 research review highlighted that expressive writing, such as sharing your deepest thoughts and feelings, may lead to benefits like fewer stress-related doctor visits, lower blood pressure, improved mood, and enhanced overall well-being.

Similarly, a 2018 study of 70 adults with medical conditions and anxiety showed that 12 weeks of writing about positive experiences, such as gratitude and reduced distress, boosted well-being. After one month, participants reported fewer symptoms of depression and anxiety, and by the second month, they experienced increased resilience.

Meditation

Meditation, widely recognized as a tool for reducing stress and anxiety, also offers benefits such as improved mood, healthier sleep patterns, and enhanced cognitive abilities. A 2014 review provided preliminary evidence that various meditation styles can enhance attention, memory, and mental sharpness in older adults. Mindfulness-based meditation programs improve sleep quality and reduce insomnia severity by helping individuals redirect racing thoughts, relax their bodies, and transition into a peaceful state conducive to rest.

A 2014 meta-analysis involving nearly 1,300 adults found that meditation significantly decreased anxiety, particularly among those with the highest anxiety levels. Additionally, a 2017 review of 45 studies showed that various meditation techniques can lower physiological markers of stress, leading to reduced anxiety levels.

An 8-week mindfulness meditation program helped individuals with generalized anxiety disorder reduce symptoms, boost positive self-statements, and improve stress management and coping skills. For workplace-related anxiety, another study revealed that employees using a mindfulness meditation app for 8 weeks experienced enhanced well-being and reduced job strain compared to a control group.

Kirtan Kriya, a meditation method that incorporates a mantra with repetitive finger movements, has shown promising results in improving cognitive performance among individuals with age-related memory loss.

Meditation is an accessible and cost-effective practice that anyone can adopt to improve mental and emotional health without requiring specialized equipment or memberships.

Balancing the mind and body is not a onetime effort, but an ongoing journey of self-care and intentional living. By adopting practices that nurture both physical health and mental clarity, you can unlock your full cognitive potential and break free from the haze of brain fog. Whether it's through nourishing nutrition, mindful movement, stress management, or restorative sleep, these strategies work together to create a foundation for lasting mental focus and well-being.

11

Finding Strength In Support

In difficult times, personal connections and support can be invaluable. Sharing experiences with others creates a sense of belonging and helps ease feelings of isolation and being overwhelmed. Whether you turn to friends, family, or a community, having a supportive network provides reassurance and encouragement, making it easier to overcome challenges and build resilience.

Building a Support Network

Building a support network is about nurturing meaningful relationships with people who can provide understanding, encouragement, and help during challenging times. These connections can include family members, close friends, coworkers, or members of groups with shared interests or similar experiences. A strong support network acts as a foundation of emotional stability, offering comfort and reassurance when life feels overwhelming.

To cultivate such a network, it is important to take an active role in reaching out to others and maintaining open, honest communication. Share your thoughts, experiences, and needs with the people you trust. Vulnerability fosters intimacy and allows others to understand how they can support you better. Similarly, being a source of encouragement and understanding for others can strengthen these bonds and create a mutual sense of reliance.

Besides self-care, seeking support groups can be immensely beneficial. Connecting with other women who are going through similar experiences can provide not only reassurance but also valuable insights. Sharing your journey with a community fosters a sense of belonging, helping to ease feelings of isolation. Through these connections, you may discover practical tips and strategies for managing your symptoms.

A well-established support network does more than provide emotional comfort; it can also bolster your resilience and equip you with the strength needed to tackle life's difficulties. It serves as a reminder that you are not alone and that together, you can navigate difficult times with greater ease and confidence.

Improve Communication

To help family members better understand your experience, it's crucial to communicate openly about what you're going through and the type of support you need. Menopause can be a complex and challenging phase, and fostering understanding within your household can make a significant difference.

Partners play an essential role during this time, yet women often exclude them from conversations about menopause. By involving your partner and candidly discussing the physical and emotional challenges you face, you can help them appreciate your experience and provide the support you need. Encouraging their participation fosters a sense of teamwork, which can strengthen your bond and ease this transition.

Similarly, children may notice changes in your behavior, mood, or energy levels, but they may not understand the reasons behind them. Taking the time to explain what menopause is and how it affects you can ease any confusion or concerns they might have. Tailoring the conversation to their age and understanding can ensure they feel involved and empathetic.

Small but meaningful actions, such as asking for help with household responsibilities like cooking, cleaning, or managing finances, can have a significant impact. These requests not only reduce your stress but also involve your family in navigating this phase together. Sharing responsibilities fosters a sense of unity and helps strengthen family bonds.

Emotional Support

Taking care of yourself is vital during this time, and prioritizing self-care can significantly affect your overall well-being. Start by practicing mindfulness or meditation, as these techniques can help calm your mind, reduce stress, and enhance your emotional resilience. Make space in your day for hobbies or activities you genuinely enjoy, as they provide a sense of fulfillment and joy and give you time to unwind. Take breaks when you feel overwhelmed; rest and downtime are essential for maintaining your energy and focus.

Seeking Professional Help

During particularly challenging times, reaching out to counselors, therapists, or medical professionals can help provide essential guidance and support. These experts can provide tailored tools, strategies, and insights to address emotional, mental, or physical struggles. Seeking help is a proactive step, equipping you with the resources needed to move forward with greater confidence and clarity.

If you find you are struggling to cope, then please seek professional help. A therapist or counselor can offer strategies to manage stress and anxiety related to cognitive changes. If your symptoms are severe or affect your daily life, consulting a doctor is important. They can rule out other potential causes and explore treatment options with you.

Support is a valuable resource when dealing with the challenges of brain fog. Turning to friends, family, or a supportive community can provide encouragement, empathy, and a sense of shared understanding. These connections help ease the emotional burden, offering strength and clarity during difficult times. Recognizing that you don't have to face these struggles alone can foster resilience and help you move forward with greater confidence.

12

Thriving At Work Despite Brain Fog

Brain fog during menopause can feel especially challenging in a professional setting, where focus, productivity, and communication are critical. A study of 351 working women (aged 40-65) revealed that 77% reported work challenges due to menopause, affecting productivity (57%) and their perceived capabilities (51%), although menopause wasn't the study's sole focus. While two-thirds of women who took part in the study desired formal menopausal policies or managerial training, less than 7% reported such requests as being in effect at their workplace.

In 2023, a United Kingdom government study examined the overall impact of menopause, although it did not specifically focus on brain fog. The result was a four-point plan that included encouraging communication, raising awareness, implementing support strategies, and sharing best practices among employers.

Even as companies work to implement menopause-related policies, your career does not have to be derailed by menopause. By managing your workload effectively and leveraging technology to your advantage, you can navigate these challenges.

Enhance Your Potential For Success

Instead of stressing about what is going wrong, which can further exacerbate the problem, there are steps you can take to help while at work.

When possible, take advantage of all breaks during the day to allow yourself to recharge and process the day's events. Even just stretching, walking up and down stairs, or sitting quietly and focusing on your briefing for five minutes can help you manage stress levels. These micro-breaks can mitigate brain and decision fatigue, allowing you to be more productive throughout the day.

Use or build a personal support network at work by connecting with an individual or a group that can support you, and if needed, provide a good laugh to reduce stress.

Optimize Your Workspace

An organized workspace can help promote focus and productivity. By keeping the space clutter-free, a clean desk can reduce the feeling of being overwhelmed. The concept of "outer order, inner calm," popularized by Gretchen Rubin in her book "Outer Order, Inner Calm: Declutter and Organize to Make More Room for Happiness," emphasizes that a tidy and organized external environment can lead to a sense of peace and calm within oneself. Our environment can significantly influence our state of mind, and by taking control of our physical space, we can create a more harmonious and serene inner world.

If you have a home office or the ability to adjust your workspace, maximize the use of natural light at your desk by positioning it near a window and using sheer curtains to soften direct sunlight if necessary. This can further help promote a calm environment. Alternatively, use layered lighting to combine ambient, task, and accent lighting, creating a balanced and adaptable lighting setup. If possible, choose calming colors like soft blues, greens, and neutrals in your office décor, and incorporate plants and artwork to enhance comfort and focus.

If you cannot adjust your surroundings, the use of noise-canceling headphones or white noise machines may help improve your focus by blocking out external sounds or reducing background noise for a more serene environment. When using headphones, be sure to use lower volume levels to protect your hearing.

Creating a Structured Routine

Brain fog often gets worse when life feels chaotic, so strong organizational tools can help you stay on track. Also, having a known schedule gives you a sense of control over your day, reducing the feeling of being scattered or directionless.

Having a set schedule promotes consistent productivity by establishing clear times for work, rest, and leisure. You can structure your day more effectively and complete important tasks without feeling overwhelmed by using digital tools such as calendar applications (apps), to-do lists, and reminder apps. Reserve time for breaks to recharge and prevent burnout. Many people find mornings are ideal for deep work, while afternoons are better suited for meetings or routine tasks.

These apps can also help break your tasks into smaller steps to avoid feeling overwhelmed and allow you to choose "focus times" during the day when you feel mentally sharper to tackle challenging tasks without interruptions.

Another potential way to ease the brain fog is by creating a "brain dump" journal, where you can list all lingering thoughts and tasks. Writing all your thoughts and tasks in one place helps declutter your mind, making it easier to focus on the present moment. With a clear mind, you can concentrate more effectively on the task at hand, thus improving overall cognitive performance. Also, knowing that you have captured all your thoughts and tasks can help reduce anxiety and stress, which are often contributors to brain fog. Journaling before bed can help clear your mind, leading to a more restful night's sleep and a fresher start the next day.

A structured routine helps organize your day, reducing mental clutter and enhancing overall clarity. It is also helpful to end your day by reviewing what you did and planning for the next day.

Managing Workload During Menopause

Taking control of your workload helps minimize stress and reduces the strain on your cognitive resources. To help reduce your brain's workload, focus on high-affected tasks and delegate tasks that do not require your expertise to team members or external support where possible. By sharing responsibilities, you lessen the mental burden on yourself, allowing for clearer thinking and better focus, while delegating tasks enables you to concentrate on high-priority activities that require your expertise, increasing overall productivity.

Practice saying "no" to unnecessary commitments that could overwhelm your schedule. With fewer commitments, you can concentrate better on the tasks at hand, leading to improved cognitive function and clarity. Also, by declining additional tasks that aren't essential, you prevent your schedule from becoming overloaded, which may reduce the feeling of being overwhelmed. When you're not spread too thin, you are more likely to make more thoughtful and informed decisions, which can contribute to a clearer mind.

Focus on one task at a time and avoid multitasking to avoid overloading your brain with too much information, which can increase the effects of brain fog. With a structured approach to your tasks, your mind stays clear and focused, allowing for better decision-making and problem-solving. By planning and prioritizing your tasks, you can manage your time more effectively and complete important tasks without unnecessary stress.

Set micro-goals and celebrate progress to stay motivated. Micro-goals break down larger tasks into manageable steps, making it easier to stay focused and clear-minded. Celebrating small successes provides a sense of accomplishment and boosts your motivation. Achieving micro-goals also reinforces your confidence in your abilities, encouraging a positive mindset.

To help prioritize your tasks, you can also use methods like the Eisenhower Matrix or the Pomodoro technique to focus on what's truly important.

The Eisenhower Matrix, also known as the Urgent-Important Matrix, is a time management tool that helps prioritize tasks based on their urgency and importance. The matrix divides tasks into four quadrants: Urgent and Important, Important but Not Urgent, Urgent but Not Important and Not Urgent and Not Important. By categorizing tasks into these quadrants, you can determine which activities to address immediately, schedule for later, delegate, or eliminate, leading to more effective time management and productivity.

Alternatively, the Pomodoro Technique is a time management method that helps improve focus and productivity by breaking work into short, focused intervals, usually 25 minutes, followed by a quick break. This breaks large projects into smaller, manageable tasks to avoid feeling overwhelmed and helps to prevent burnout by incorporating regular breaks. Using online project management tools to visualize each step of your projects can significantly reduce brain fog and offer multiple benefits. These tools can help break down complex projects into clear, manageable steps, reducing mental clutter and making it easier to understand what needs to be done. You can also use these tools to prioritize tasks and allocate your time effectively, thus meeting deadlines without unnecessary stress.

Some apps, like ClickUp, Monday.com, Asana and Trello, allow you to visualize your tasks and timelines, helping you stay organized and keep track of your progress. This can minimize the feeling of being overwhelmed. These and similar apps can also assist you in assigning tasks within the tool, which helps reduce mental clutter and improve overall productivity, ultimately easing brain fog.

13

A Clearer Path Ahead

One of the most comforting truths about experiencing brain fog during menopause is that it is incredibly common, even if it feels deeply personal. Millions of women face these same challenges, yet many feel alone because people don't discuss menopausal brain fog enough.

Cultural stigma surrounding aging and menopause often make women hesitant to discuss their symptoms. In an article from May 2024, 28 celebrities shared their menopause journeys. Out of these 28 women, only one—Oprah Winfrey—mentioned that brain fog was affecting her concentration. This lack of public acknowledgment of this symptom creates a false sense of isolation among women, making it appear you are the only one fumbling through your sentences or forgetting why you walked into a room.

Understanding that brain fog has a biological basis allows you to approach it with a proactive mindset. Brain fog occurs because your body is responding to a significant hormonal overhaul. This is not a reflection of your intelligence or abilities; rather, it is about how your brain is adapting to a new hormonal landscape. By acknowledging this, you are not showing weakness or failure. Recognizing this can help you stop blaming yourself and start focusing on strategies to clear the fog.

Combine the lack of public awareness with it occurring when you are likely to experience family issues, aging parents, college-aged kids, and career challenges either through battling with multiple tasks or competing with the younger generation, it's no surprise then that your brain feels overloaded and so you end up with the mental fuzziness that is brain fog.

Open conversations about symptoms, even those that are not immediately apparent to others, can help normalize the experience and foster understanding. Women should feel empowered to share what they're going through with trusted friends, family, or colleagues, if comfortable, to build a supportive network. Similarly, raising awareness about the less visible aspects of menopause can help create more compassionate and informed environments, both at home and in the workplace.

Surround yourself with people who understand and uplift you. Lean on friends, family, or colleagues when you need encouragement or practical help. The fog may linger, but it does not have to limit you. You have the tools, strength, and resilience to create a life of clarity, joy, and fulfillment. Clinical psychologists recommend focusing on the benefits of menopause by focusing on yourself while no longer having to deal with your menstrual cycle.

The good news is that while brain fog can feel overwhelming, it is also manageable. Recognizing its effects is the first step toward reclaiming control. Remind yourself that menopause is a phase, not a permanent state. See it as a chapter in your life, not the entire story. Focus on what you can control rather than dwelling on frustrations. Be kind to yourself and acknowledge that this is a phase, not a flaw, to ease the emotional toll and empower you to adapt.

Brain fog during menopause may feel like an uphill battle, but the journey becomes easier when you remember two things: it is not all in your head, and you do not have to face it alone.

Menopause brain fog does not define you; it is just one part of your journey.

14

The Brain Fog Toolkit

When brain fog hits, it can be frustrating and disorienting. This quick guide provides simple, actionable strategies to help clear the haze and regain mental clarity. Use these techniques whenever you need a mental reset.

Mindset & Quick Coping Strategies

- Pause and breathe: Take five deep, slow breaths to oxygenate your brain and reduce stress.

- Name it to tame it: Acknowledge, *"This is brain fog, not me,"* to detach from frustration.

- Use humor: Laughing at forgetfulness helps ease tension and promotes a positive mindset.

- Reframe expectations: Give yourself permission to slow down and focus on one thing at a time.

Brain-Boosting Nutrition

- Hydrate! Drink a glass of water as dehydration worsens brain fog.

- Snack smart: Choose brain-friendly foods like nuts, seeds, and berries for a quick mental boost.

- Limit sugar and caffeine: Avoid processed sugar and excessive caffeine, which can lead to energy crashes.

- Eat healthy fats: Incorporate avocados, salmon, and olive oil to support cognitive function.

Move Your Body, Wake Up Your Brain

- Stretch or move: A quick two-minute stretch or walk improves circulation and brain function.

- Step outside: Natural sunlight helps reset your brain and improve alertness.

- Try deep breathing exercises: Box breathing (inhale for 4 seconds, hold for 4, exhale for 4, hold for 4) helps reset focus.

- Listen to music: Upbeat or calming tunes can stimulate cognitive function and enhance mood.

Organizational Hacks

- Keep a brain fog journal: Track symptoms, triggers, and what helps clear your mind.

- Use reminders: Set phone alarms, write sticky notes, or use a planner for important tasks.

- Follow the "one thing at a time" rule: Multitasking can worsen brain fog, so it is best to focus on single tasks.

- Break tasks into steps: Simplify overwhelming tasks into smaller, more manageable pieces.

Rest & Recovery

- Take a 10-minute break: Step away from mental strain to recharge.

- Prioritize sleep: Aim for consistent, high-quality rest in a dark, cool, and quiet space.

- Try a quick nap: A 20–30-minute power nap can refresh your mind without causing grogginess.

- Reduce blue light exposure: Limit screen time before bed to improve sleep quality and brain function.

Final Thought

Brain fog can feel overwhelming, but small, intentional actions can make a big difference. When in doubt, hydrate, breathe, move, and be kind to yourself. With the right tools, you can navigate the fog and reclaim mental clarity!

Thank You

Dear Reader,

Thank you so much for taking the time to read my book. Your support means the world to me. If you found value in this book, I'd be incredibly grateful if you could take a few minutes to leave a review on Amazon or Goodreads. Your feedback not only helps me improve, but also helps other readers discover the book. Whether it's a few words or a detailed review, your voice matters and makes a big difference!

Warm regards, R.D. Bennett

Resources

Chapter 1: Unlocking The Path To Clarity

- *Brain fog*. (n.d.). https://www.letstalkmenopause.org/our-articles/brain-fog

- Suszynski, M. (2011, July 19). Menopause and sweating. WebMD. https://www.webmd.com/menopause/features/menopause-sweating-11

- Ferrari, N. (2020, August 14). Menopause-related hot flashes and night sweats can last for years. Harvard Health. https://www.health.harvard.edu/blog/menopause-related-hot-flashes-night-sweats-can-last-years-201502237745

- Loss of libido symptom information. (2020, October 15). Menopause Now. https://www.menopausenow.com/loss-libido

- Kennedy, Q., PhD. (2023, July 6). Brain fog due to menopause is more common than many people think. *Psychology Today*.

- https://www.psychologytoday.com/us/blog/aging-and-cognition/202306/its-not-alzheimers-disease-its-perimenopause

- Levine, B. (2024, August 27). What is vaginal dryness? Symptoms, causes, diagnosis, treatment, and prevention. EverydayHealth.com.
https://www.everydayhealth.com/vaginal-dryness/guide/

- Brighten, J. (2024, October 3). The connection between brain fog and hormone imbalance. Dr. Jolene Brighten. https://drbrighten.com/brain-fog-and-hormonal-imbalance/#:~:text=Let%E2%80%99s%20start%20with%20the

- Menopause - Society for Women's Health Research. (2024, November 8). Society for Women's Health Research. https://swhr.org/health_focus_area/menopause/

Chapter 2: Unraveling The Mystery Of Brain Fog

- Coslov, N., Richardson, M. K., & Woods, N. F. (2024). "Not feeling like myself" in perimenopause — what does it mean? Observations from the Women Living Better survey. *Menopause the Journal of the North American Menopause Society.* https://doi.org/10.1097/gme.0000000000002339

- Hogervorst, E., Donnell D, E., & Hardy, R. (n.d.). *Menopause: HRT's brain-protecting effect may be overstated.* The Conversation. https://theconversation.com/menopause-hrts-brain-protecting-effect-may-be-overstated-1824182449

- Karlamangla, A. S., Lachman, M. E., Han, W., Huang, M., & Greendale, G. A. (2017). Evidence for Cognitive aging in midlife Women: Study of Women's health across the nation. *PLoS ONE, 12*(1), e0169008. https://doi.org/10.1371/journal.pone.0169008
- Maki, P. M., & Jaff, N. G. (2024). Menopause and brain fog: how to counsel and treat midlife women. *Menopause the Journal of the North American Menopause Society, 31*(7), 647–649. https://doi.org/10.1097/gme.0000000000002382
- NeuroLaunch.com. (2024, August 26). *Sleep deprivation and brain fog: the hidden connection.* https://neurolaunch.com/can-lack-of-sleep-cause-brain-fog/
- Salamon, M. (2022, June 1). *Menopause and brain fog: What's the link?* Harvard Health. https://www.health.harvard.edu/womens-health/menopause-and-brain-fog-whats-the-link
- Zhu, C., Arunogiri, S., Thomas, E. H. X., Li, Q., Kulkarni, J., & Gurvich, C. (2024). The development and evaluation of a fact sheet resource for women managing menopausal-related cognitive complaints. *Menopause the Journal of the North American Menopause Society.* https://doi.org/10.1097/gme.0000000000002434
- Zhu, C., Thomas, E. H., Li, Q., Arunogiri, S., Thomas, N., & Gurvich, C. (2023). Evaluation of the Everyday Memory Questionnaire-Revised in a menopausal population: understanding the brain fog during menopause. *Menopause the Journal of the North American Menopause Society, 30*(11),

1147–1156.
https://doi.org/10.1097/gme.0000000000002256

Chapter 3: The Ripple Effects Of Brain Fog

- *Age variation in the divorce rate, 1990 & 2021. (n.d.-b). Bowling Green State University.* https://www.bgsu.edu/ncfmr/resources/data/family-profiles/westrick-payne-lin-age-variation-divorce-rate-1990-2021-fp-23-16.html

- Jennifer Sauer, Laura Mehegan, Alicia Williams, Aisha Bonner-Cozad, Cheryl Lampkin, Monica Ekman, The Economic Impact Of Menopause: A Multimode Research Project, *Innovation in Aging*, Volume 7, Issue Supplement_1, December 2023, Page 587, https://doi.org/10.1093/geroni/igad104.1921

- Faubion, S. S., Enders, F., Hedges, M. S., Chaudhry, R., Kling, J. M., Shufelt, C. L., Saadedine, M., Mara, K., Griffin, J. M., & Kapoor, E. (2023). Impact of menopause symptoms on women in the workplace. *Mayo Clinic Proceedings*, 98(6), 833–845. https://doi.org/10.1016/j.mayocp.2023.02.025

- *Shattering the Silence about Menopause: 12-Month Progress Report. (2024, March 8). GOV.UK.* https://www.gov.uk/government/publications/shattering-the-silence-about-menopause-12-month-progress-report/shattering-the-silence-about-menopause-12-month-progress-report

- Anne Hayes. (n.d.). Lifting the second glass ceiling. In *BSI*. https://www.bsigroup.com/globalassets/localfiles/en-

- gb/topics/prioritizing-people/glass-ceiling/bsi-sgc-whitepaper.pdf.

- Kirsty. (2022, September 9). *Menopause and perimenopause impact on divorce and separation in midlife.* Leiper Gupta Family
Lawyers Reading, Divorce Solicitors Berkshire. https://lgfamilylawyers.co.uk/impact-of-menopause-on-divorce-and-separation/

- Mayer, K. (2024, January 10). Employers are turning to a new perk: menopause
benefits. *SHRM.* https://www.shrm.org/topics-tools/news/benefits-compensation/menopause-benefits-new-workplace-trend

- Schurman, B., & Fadal, T. (2024, January 11). *How companies can support employees experiencing menopause.* Harvard Business Review. https://hbr.org/2024/01/how-companies-can-support-employees-experiencing-menopause

- America, B. O. (2024, January 25). *Menopause in the Workplace Report: Impact, facts, statistics.* Bank of America. https://business.bofa.com/en-us/content/workplace-benefits/menopause-in-the-workplace.html

- Johnson, S. (2024, March 21). *Menopause and Divorce: Is there a Link? (+ 5 Tips for Coping).* SimplyMenopause. https://simplymenopause.net/menopause-and-divorce/

- Menopause Friendly Accreditation, Independent Panel. (2024, July 17). *Menopause Friendly Employer Awards 2023.*

- Menopause Friendly UK. https://menopausefriendly.co.uk/mfea-2024/mfea23/

- NeuroLaunch.com. (2024, August 20). *Brain Fog at work: Strategies to Boost Productivity and Mental Clarity.* https://neurolaunch.com/brain-fog-at-work/

- Department for Work and Pensions. (2024, October 17). Women's health campaigner Mariella Frostrup appointed as Government Menopause Employment Ambassador. *GOV. UK.* https://www.gov.uk/government/news/womens-health-campaigner-mariella-frostrup-appointed-as-government-menopause-employment-ambassador

- Thapliyal, A. (2024, October 18). *Progress, but not Enough: Why there is an Urgent Need for Menopause Inclusivity in Workplaces.* All Things Talent. https://allthingstalent.org/progress-but-not-enough-why-there-is-an-urgent-need-for-menopause-inclusivity-in-workplaces/2024/10/18/

- Bieber, C., JD. (2024, November 20). *Revealing divorce statistics in 2025.* Forbes Advisor. https://www.forbes.com/advisor/legal/divorce/divorce-statistics/#sources_section

Chapter 4: The Brain and Cognitive Function: A Deeper Look

- Helmenstine, A. (2025, March 16). *Parts of the brain and their functions.* Science Notes and Projects. https://sciencenotes.org/parts-of-the-brain-and-their-functions/

- Martin, L. (2023, February 10). *What to know about the brain.* https://www.medicalnewstoday.com/articles/brain

- MSc, O. G. (2023, November 9). *Parts of the Brain: Anatomy, Structure & Functions.* Simply Psychology. https://www.simplypsychology.org/anatomy-of-the-brain.html

- Professional, C. C. M. (2025, January 28). *Brain.* Cleveland Clinic. https://my.clevelandclinic.org/health/body/22638-brain.

Chapter 5: Cognitive Function: Understanding the Brain's Interactions and Needs

- Denno, P., Zhao, S., Husain, M., & Hampshire, A. (2025). Defining brain fog across medical conditions. *Trends in Neurosciences.* https://doi.org/10.1016/j.tins.2025.01.003

- Falde, N. (2024, April 19). *Beginners guide to understanding the cognitive functions.* True You Journal. https://www.truity.com/blog/beginners-guide-understanding-mbti-cognitive-functions

- Warner, D. (2024, June 20). *What to know about cognitive functioning.* https://www.medicalnewstoday.com/articles/cognitive-functioning

- Professional, C. C. M. (2024, December 19). *Neurotransmitters.* Cleveland Clinic. https://my.clevelandclinic.org/health/articles/22513-neurotransmitters

- Professional, C. C. M. (2024, December 19). *Brain fog*. Cleveland Clinic. https://my.clevelandclinic.org/health/symptoms/brain-fog

Chapter 6: Hormones And Brain Fog: The Missing Link?

- Haufe, A., & Leeners, B. (2023). Sleep disturbances across a woman's lifespan: What is the role of reproductive hormones? Journal of the Endocrine Society, 7(5). https://doi.org/10.1210/jendso/bvad036

- Grainger, S. (n.d.). Testosterone and Women - Australasian Menopause Society. https://www.menopause.org.au/health-info/resources/testosterone-and-women

- Davis, S. (n.d.). Don't believe the hype. Menopausal women don't all need to check – or increase – their testosterone levels. The Conversation. https://theconversation.com/dont-believe-the-hype-menopausal-women-dont-all-need-to-check-or-increase-their-testosterone-levels-209516

- Grainger, S. (n.d.-b). Testosterone use in women - Australasian Menopause Society. https://www.menopause.org.au/hp/gp-hp-resources/testosterone-use-in-women

- Davis, S. R., Baber, R., Panay, N., Bitzer, J., Perez, S. C., Islam, R. M., Kaunitz, A. M., Kingsberg, S. A., Lambrinoudaki, I., Liu, J., Parish, S. J., Pinkerton, J., Rymer, J., Simon, J. A., Vignozzi, L., & Wierman, M. E. (2019). Global Consensus Position Statement on the Use of

- Testosterone therapy for Women. *Climacteric, 22*(5), 429–434. https://doi.org/10.1080/13697137.2019.1637079

- Gibson, C. J., Thurston, R. C., & Matthews, K. A. (2016). Cortisol dysregulation is associated with daily diary-reported hot flashes among midlife women. *Clinical Endocrinology, 85*(4), 645–651. https://doi.org/10.1111/cen.13076

- Johns Hopkins Medical. (n.d.). Do menopausal women have an increased risk of cardiovascular disease? Retrieved December 6, 2024, from https://www.hopkinsmedicine.org/health/conditions-and-diseases/menopause-and-the-heart

- Heart failure, atrial fibrillation & coronary heart disease linked to cognitive impairment. (n.d.). American Heart Association. https://newsroom.heart.org/news/heart-failure-atrial-fibrillation-coronary-heart-disease-linked-to-cognitive-impairment

- DeAngelis, T. (n.d.). Menopause can be rough. Psychology is here to help. https://www.apa.org/monitor/2023/09/easing-transition-into-menopause

- Mosconi, L., Nerattini, M., Matthews, D. C., Jett, S., Andy, C., Williams, S., Yepez, C. B., Zarate, C., Carlton, C., Fauci, F., Ajila, T., Pahlajani, S., Andrews, R., Pupi, A., Ballon, D., Kelly, J., Osborne, J. R., Nehmeh, S., Fink, M., Brinton, R. D. (2024). In vivo brain estrogen receptor density by neuroendocrine aging and relationships with cognition and symptomatology. *Scientific Reports, 14*(1). https://doi.org/10.1038/s41598-024-62820-7

- Admin, W. (2021, September 4). The Effects of Hormones on Brain Health — Women's Brain Health Initiative. Women's Brain Health Initiative. https://womensbrainhealth.org/think-tank/better-thinking/the-effects-of-hormones-on-brain-health

- Charity, M. (2021, October 21). Brain fog. The Menopause Charity. https://www.themenopausecharity.org/2021/10/21/brain-fog/

- Levine, H. (2023, June 29). *How menopause messes with your brain*. AARP. https://www.aarp.org/health/brain-health/info-2021/menopause-brain-fog.html?msockid=1206e760cd3366970868e838cc846793

- Mfa, R. J. S. (2024, January 5). What to know about progesterone therapy for menopause. Healthline. https://www.healthline.com/health/progesterone-for-menopause#what-it-is

- Mayo Clinic Press. (2024, March 27). *Women's Health - Mayo Clinic Press*. https://mcpress.mayoclinic.org/women-health/#:~:text=After%20menopause%2C%20changes%20in%20your%20hormone%20levels%20can,you%20have%20a%20higher%20risk%20of%20diabetes%20complications

- Christiansen, S. (2024, March 29). *How progesterone promotes brain health*. Verywell Health. https://www.verywellhealth.com/progesterone-and-brain-health-4589255

- Ceboniboykin. (2024, April 17). *Testosterone — Not just for men*. Mayo Clinic Press. https://mcpress.mayoclinic.org/women-health/testosterone-not-just-for-men/

- Professional, C. C. M. (2024, May 1). Thyroid hormone. Cleveland Clinic. https://my.clevelandclinic.org/health/articles/22391-thyroid-hormone

- Professional, C. C. M. (2024, May 1). Cortisol. Cleveland Clinic. https://my.clevelandclinic.org/health/articles/22187-cortisol

- Menopause. (2024, June 25). Cleveland Clinic. https://my.clevelandclinic.org/health/diseases/21841-menopause

- Clinic, C. (2024, June 25). How estrogen supports heart health. Cleveland Clinic. https://health.clevelandclinic.org/estrogen-and-heart-health

- Clinic, C. (2024, July 9). Estrogen: What it does and 5 Benefits. Cleveland Clinic. https://health.clevelandclinic.org/what-does-estrogen-do

- Your brain and diabetes. (2024, July 16). Diabetes. https://www.cdc.gov/diabetes/diabetes-complications/effects-of-diabetes-brain.html

- Chesak, J. (2024, July 17). Your brain might try to stockpile estrogen during Menopause—And it could explain brain fog. *Verywell Health*. https://www.verywellhealth.com/causes-of-menopause-brain-fog-8675607#citation-3

- Nd, M. J. (2024, August 9). Do you have a menopause brain? Women's Health Network. https://www.womenshealthnetwor

- k.com/menopause-and-perimenopause/do-you-have-menopause-brain/

- Marcin, A. (2024, October 21). What causes menopause brain fog,
  and how is it treated? Healthline. https://www.healthline.com/health/menopause/menopause-brain-fog#prevention

- How perimenopause and menopause affect the brain. (2024, November 8). https://www.brainandlife.org/articles/perimenopause-menopause-affect-brain

- American Thyroid Association. (2025, February 17). *Vol 18 Issue 2 P.3-4 | American Thyroid Association.* https://www.thyroid.org/patient-thyroid-information/ct-for-patients/february-2025/vol-18-issue-2-p-3-4/

- Admin, W. (2021b, September 4). *The Effects of hormones on Brain Health — Women's Brain Health Initiative.* Women's Brain Health Initiative. https://womensbrainhealth.org/think-tank/better-thinking/the-effects-of-hormones-on-brain-health

Chapter 7: Fueling Mental Clarity

- Cui, C., Birru, R. L., Snitz, B. E., Ihara, M., Kakuta, C., Lopresti, B. J., Aizenstein, H. J., Lopez, O. L., Mathis, C. A., Miyamoto, Y., Kuller, L. H., & Sekikawa, A. (2019). Effects of soy isoflavones on cognitive function: a systematic review and meta-analysis of randomized controlled trials. *Nutrition Reviews, 78*(2), 134–144. https://doi.org/10.1093/nutrit/nuz050

- Henderson, V., St John, J., Hodis, H., Kono, N., McCleary, C., Franke, A., & Mack, W. (2012). Long-term soy isoflavone supplementation and cognition in women. *Neurology*, *78*(23), 1841–1848. https://doi.org/10.1212/wnl.0b013e318258f822

- Dighriri, I. M., Alsubaie, A. M., Hakami, F. M., Hamithi, D. M., Alshekh, M. M., Khobrani, F. A., Dalak, F. E., Hakami, A. A., Alsueaadi, E. H., Alsaawi, L. S., Alshammari, S. F., Alqahtani, A. S., Alawi, I. A., Aljuaid, A. A., & Tawhari, M. Q. (2022). Effects of omega-3 polyunsaturated fatty acids on brain functions: a systematic review. *Cureus*. https://doi.org/10.7759/cureus.30091

- Raymond-Lezman, J. R., & Riskin, S. I. (2023). Benefits and risks of sun exposure to maintain adequate vitamin D levels. *Cureus*. https://doi.org/10.7759/cureus.38578

- Clarkson, T. B., Utian, W. H., Barnes, S., Gold, E. B., Basaria, S. S., Aso, T., Kronenberg, F., Frankenfeld, C. L., Cline, J. M., Landgren, B., Gallagher, J. C., Weaver, C. M., Hodis, H. N., Brinton, R. D., & Maki, P. M. (2011). The role of soy isoflavones in menopausal health. *Menopause the Journal of the North American Menopause Society*, *18*(7), 732–753. https://doi.org/10.1097/gme.0b013e31821fc8e0

- Sievert, L. L., Obermeyer, C. M., & Price, K. (2006). Determinants of hot flashes and night sweats. *Annals of Human Biology*, *33*(1), 4–16. https://doi.org/10.1080/03014460500421338

- Schilling, C., Gallicchio, L., Miller, S. R., Langenberg, P., Zacur, H., & Flaws, J. A. (2007). Current alcohol use, hormone levels, and hot flashes in midlife women. *Fertility and Sterility*, *87*(6), 1483–1486. https://doi.org/10.1016/j.fertnstert.2006.11.033

- *Alcohol, hormones, and postmenopausal women.* (1998). PubMed. https://pubmed.ncbi.nlm.nih.gov/15706794/

- Lakhan, R., Sharma, M., Batra, K., & Beatty, F. B. (2021). The role of vitamin E in Slowing down mild Cognitive Impairment: A Narrative review. *Healthcare*, *9*(11), 1573. https://doi.org/10.3390/healthcare9111573

- Ferreira, A., Neves, P., & Gozzelino, R. (2019). Multilevel affects of Iron in the Brain: The Cross Talk between Neurophysiological Mechanisms, Cognition, and Social Behavior. *Pharmaceuticals*, *12*(3), 126. https://doi.org/10.3390/ph12030126

- Ask a Professor: Is zinc good for your memory? | Colgate Magazine

- Scheiber, I. F., Mercer, J. F., & Dringen, R. (2014). Metabolism and functions of copper in brain. *Progress in Neurobiology*, *116*, 33–57. https://doi.org/10.1016/j.pneurobio.2014.01.002

- Cirino, E. (2020, November 30). *Can you drink during menopause?* Healthline. https://www.healthline.com/health/menopause/alcohol#research-on-alcohol-and-menopause

- Godman, H. (2022, June 1). *Protein intake associated with less cognitive decline.* Harvard Health. https://www.health.harvard.edu/mind-and-mood/protein-intake-associated-with-less-cognitive-decline

- Rd, R. a. M. (2022, June 13). *Can certain nutrient deficiencies cause brain fog?* Healthline. https://www.healthline.com/nutrition/can-not-enough-nutrients-cause-brain-fog#fa-qs

- Rusbatch, S. (2022, September 1). *Sarah Rusbatch – Drinking alcohol affects menopause in 5 alarming ways – what to watch out for — Sarah Rusbatch | Sobriety & Grey Area Drinking Coach, Speaker.* Sarah Rusbatch | Sobriety & Grey Area Drinking Coach, Speaker. https://sarahrusbatch.com/blog/5-alarming-ways-drinking-impacts-menopause

- PharmD, S. M. (2022, October 24). Dehydration and brain fog: what you need to know. *Neuro Section9.* https://www.neurosection9.com/dehydration/#:~:text=Dehydration%20can%20lead%20to%20all%20sorts%20of%20problems%2C,to%20stay%20hydrated%20and%20avoid%20dehydration-related%20brain%20fog

- Rd, R. a. M. (2023, February 14). *Zinc supplements: benefits, dosage, and side effects.* Healthline. https://www.healthline.com/nutrition/zinc-supplements#benefits

- Velasco Hames, M. (2023, May 5). Mayo Clinic Minute: Why alcohol and Menopause can be a dangerous mix. newsnetwork.mayoclinic.org. Retrieved December 6, 2024, from https://newsnetwork.mayoclinic.org/discussion/mayo-

- clinic-minute-why-alcohol-and-menopause-can-be-a-dangerous-mix/

- Levine, H. (2023, June 29). *How menopause messes with your brain.* AARP. https://www.aarp.org/health/brain-health/info-2021/menopause-brain-fog.html?msockid=1206e760cd3366970868e838cc846793

- Rd, K. P. P. (2023, July 25). *How omega-3 fish oil affects your brain and mental health.* Healthline. https://www.healthline.com/nutrition/omega-3-fish-oil-for-brain-health

- Kellot, T. (2024, August 20). What vitamins are good for brain fog? *Science of mind.* https://scienceofmind.org/what-vitamins-are-good-for-brain-fog/

- NeuroLaunch.com. (2024, October 3). *Dehydration and brain fog: the surprising connection and how to Combat it.* https://neurolaunch.com/can-dehydration-cause-brain-fog/

- NeuroLaunch.com. (2024, October 22). *NeuroLaunch.com: Where grey matter matters.* https://neurolaunch.com/

- Powell, J. (2024, November 7). *Straight talk about soy - the nutrition source.* The Nutrition Source. https://nutritionsource.hsph.harvard.edu/soy/

- Admin. (2024, November 7). *Protein - the nutrition source.* The Nutrition Source. https://nutritionsource.hsph.harvard.edu/what-should-you-eat/protein/

- Christiansen, S. (2024, November 24). *Isoflavones*. Verywell Health. https://www.verywellhealth.com/isoflavones-benefits-side-effects-dosage-and-interactions-4687017

- Rd, J. K. M. (2024, December 10). *6 Best Evidence-Based Supplements for Brain Fog*. Healthline. https://www.healthline.com/nutrition/vitamins-for-brain-fog

- Randall, P. (2025, January 20). *How minerals can improve focus and memory*. Trace Minerals. https://www.traceminerals.com/blogs/lifestyle/how-to-get-rid-of-brain-fog-with-minerals

- Perlmutter, A., MD. (2025, February 24). Research suggests diverse causes and potential tools for this common condition. *Psychology Today*. https://www.psychologytoday.com/us/blog/the-modern-brain/202502/the-top-causes-of-brain-fog?msockid=1206e760cd3366970868e838cc846793.

Chapter 8: Balancing Mind And Body For A Clearer You

- Grindler, N. M., & Santoro, N. F. (2015). Menopause and exercise. *Menopause the Journal of the North American Menopause Society*, *22*(12), 1351–1358. https://doi.org/10.1097/gme.0000000000000536

- Sydora, B. C., Turner, C., Malley, A., Davenport, M., Yuksel, N., Shandro, T., & Ross, S. (2020). Can walking exercise programs improve health for women in menopause transition and postmenopausal? Findings from a scoping review. *Menopause the Journal of the North American Menopause Society*, *27*(8), 952–963. https://doi.org/10.1097/gme.0000000000001554

- Masmoudi, K., Chaari, F., Waer, F. B., Rebai, H., & Sahli, S. (2024). A single session of slow-paced breathing improved cognitive functions and postural control among middle-aged women: a randomized single blinded controlled trial. *Menopause the Journal of the North American Menopause Society.* https://doi.org/10.1097/gme.0000000000002470

- Sternfeld, B., Guthrie, K. A., Ensrud, K. E., LaCroix, A. Z., Larson, J. C., Dunn, A. L., Anderson, G. L., Seguin, R. A., Carpenter, J. S., Newton, K. M., Reed, S. D., Freeman, E. W., Cohen, L. S., Joffe, H., Roberts, M., & Caan, B. J. (2013). Efficacy of exercise for menopausal symptoms. *Menopause the Journal of the North American Menopause Society, 21*(4), 330–338. https://doi.org/10.1097/gme.0b013e31829e4089

- Lynne. (2024, January 30). *Managing Menopause Brain Fog with Quick Cognitive Exercises.* Menopause Network. https://menopausenetwork.org/managing-menopause-brain-fog-with-quick-cognitive-exercises/

- Storr, K. (2024, September 11). *10 tips for parenting during the menopause, according to doctors (and mums).* GoodTo. https://www.goodto.com/wellbeing/parenting-during-menopause.

- NeuroLaunch.com. (2024, October 2). *Menopause brain fog: causes, symptoms, and effective management Strategies.* https://neurolaunch.com/menopause-brain-fog/

Chapter 9: Navigating the Emotional Journey of Brain Fog

- Smyth, J. M., Johnson, J. A., Auer, B. J., Lehman, E., Talamo, G., & Sciamanna, C. N. (2018). Online Positive Affect Journaling in the Improvement of Mental Distress and Well-Being in General medical patients with Elevated Anxiety Symptoms: a preliminary randomized controlled trial. *JMIR Mental Health*, *5*(4), e11290. https://doi.org/10.2196/11290

- Pascoe, M. C., Thompson, D. R., Jenkins, Z. M., & Ski, C. F. (2017). Mindfulness mediates the physiological markers of stress: Systematic review and meta-analysis. *Journal of Psychiatric Research*, *95*, 156–178. https://doi.org/10.1016/j.jpsychires.2017.08.004

- Hoge, E. A., Bui, E., Marques, L., Metcalf, C. A., Morris, L. K., Robinaugh, D. J., Worthington, J. J., Pollack, M. H., & Simon, N. M. (2013). Randomized controlled trial of mindfulness meditation for generalized anxiety disorder. *The Journal of Clinical Psychiatry*, *74*(08), 786–792. https://doi.org/10.4088/jcp.12m08083

- Orme-Johnson, D. W., & Barnes, V. A. (2013). Effects of the Transcendental Meditation Technique on trait Anxiety: A Meta-Analysis of Randomized Controlled Trials. *The Journal of Alternative and Complementary Medicine*, *20*(5), 330–341. https://doi.org/10.1089/acm.2013.0204

- Bostock, S., Crosswell, A. D., Prather, A. A., & Steptoe, A. (2018). Mindfulness on-the-go: Effects of a mindfulness meditation app on work stress and well-being. *Journal of*

- *Occupational Health Psychology, 24*(1), 127–138. https://doi.org/10.1037/ocp0000118

- Khalsa, D. S. (2015). Stress, meditation, and Alzheimer's Disease Prevention: Where the evidence stands. *Journal of Alzheimer S Disease, 48*(1), 1–12. https://doi.org/10.3233/jad-142766

- Gard, T., Hölzel, B. K., & Lazar, S. W. (2014). The potential effects of meditation on age-related cognitive decline: a systematic review. *Annals of the New York Academy of Sciences, 1307*(1), 89–103. https://doi.org/10.1111/nyas.12348

- Thorpe, M., MD PhD. (2024, August 15). *How meditation benefits your mind and body.* Healthline. https://www.healthline.com/nutrition/12-benefits-of-meditation

- Self-Compassion. (2024, August 20). *Exploring the meaning of Self-Compassion and its importance.* https://self-compassion.org/what-is-self-compassion/

- Ms, M. T. (2024, November 12). *6 Journaling benefits and how to start right now.* Healthline. *https://www.healthline.com/health/benefits-of-journaling*

- Self-Compassion. (2025, February 5). *Self-Compassion by Kristin Neff: Join the community now.* https://self-compassion.org/

Chapter 11- Thriving Professionally Through The Haze

- Alzueta, E., Menghini, L., Volpe, L., Baker, F. C., Garnier, A., Sarrel, P. M., & De Zambotti, M. (2024). Navigating menopause at work: a preliminary study about challenges and support systems. *Menopause the Journal of the North American Menopause Society, 31*(4), 258–265. https://doi.org/10.1097/gme.0000000000002333

- Collins, B. (2020, March 3). *The Pomodoro technique explained.* Forbes. https://www.forbes.com/sites/bryancollinseurope/2020/03/03/the-pomodoro-technique/

- NeuroLaunch.com. (2024, August 20). *Brain Fog at work: Strategies to Boost Productivity and Mental Clarity.* https://neurolaunch.com/brain-fog-at-work/

- SPS Academic Resource Center. (n.d.-b). *The Eisenhower Matrix.* https://sps.columbia.edu/sites/default/files/2023-08/Eisenhower%20Matrix.pdf

Chapter 12: A Clearer Path Ahead

- Manzella, S. (2024, July 17). 26 celebrities who have gotten real about going through perimenopause & menopause. SheKnows. https://www.sheknows.com/health-and-wellness/slideshow/2658982/celebrities-going-through-menopause-perimenopause/

Other Books By R. D. Bennett

Find other books by R. D. Bennett on any of the following websites and at major book retailers:

www.rd-bennett.com

www.snowhillamerica.com

ABOUT THE AUTHOR

R. D. Bennett is a nonfiction writer based in Virginia, where she lives with her husband, daughter, and two lovable dogs. With a passion for learning and a deep interest in topics that inspire and support others, she brings a fresh perspective. Embracing a newfound joy for writing, she is excited to connect with readers and grow with each project.

www.ingramcontent.com/pod-product-compliance
Lightning Source LLC
Chambersburg PA
CBHW060519030426
42337CB00015B/1948